Thyroid and Parathyroid Imaging

Editors

SALMAAN AHMED
JAMES MATTHEW DEBNAM

NEUROIMAGING CLINICS
OF NORTH AMERICA

www.neuroimaging.theclinics.com

Consulting Editor
SURESH K. MUKHERJI

August 2021 • Volume 31 • Number 3

ELSEVIER

1600 John F. Kennedy Boulevard • Suite 1800 • Philadelphia, Pennsylvania, 19103-2899

http://www.neuroimaging.theclinics.com

NEUROIMAGING CLINICS OF NORTH AMERICA Volume 31, Number 3
August 2021 ISSN 1052-5149, ISBN 13: 978-0-323-79850-1

Editor: John Vassallo (j.vassallo@elsevier.com)
Developmental Editor: Karen Solomon

Neuroimaging Clinics of North America (ISSN 1052-5149) is published quarterly by Elsevier Inc., 360 Park Avenue South, New York, NY 10010-1710. Months of issue are February, May, August, and November. Business and editorial offices: 1600 John F. Kennedy Blvd., Suite 1800, Philadelphia, PA 19103-2899. Business and editorial offices: 6277 Sea Harbor Drive, Orlando, FL 32887-4800. Periodicals postage paid at New York, NY, and additional mailing offices. Subscription prices are USD 397 per year for US individuals, USD 918 per year for US institutions, USD 100 per year for US students and residents, USD 465 per year for Canadian individuals, USD 959 per year for Canadian institutions, USD 541 per year for international individuals, USD 959 per year for international institutions, USD 100 per year for Canadian students and residents and USD 260 per year for foreign students and residents. To receive student/resident rate, orders must be accompanied by name of affiliated institution, date of term, and the *signature* of program/residency coordinator on institution letterhead. Orders will be billed at individual rate until proof of status is received. Foreign air speed delivery is included in all *Clinics* subscription prices. All prices are subject to change without notice. POSTMASTER: Send address changes to *Neuroimaging Clinics of North America*, Elsevier Health Sciences Division, Subscription **Customer Service, 3251 Riverport Lane, Maryland Heights, MO 63043. Telephone: 1-800-654-2452 (U.S. and Canada); 314-447-8871 (outside U.S. and Canada). Fax: 314-447-8029. E-mail: journalscustomerservice-usa@elsevier.com (for print support); journalsonlinesupport-usa@elsevier.com (for online support).**

Reprints. For copies of 100 or more of articles in this publication, please contact the Commercial Reprints Department, Elsevier Inc., 360 Park Avenue South, New York, NY 10010-1710. Tel.: 212-633-3874; Fax: 212-633-3820; E-mail: reprints@elsevier.com.

Neuroimaging Clinics of North America is covered by *Excerpta Medical/EMBASE,* the RSNA Index of Imaging Literature, *MEDLINE/PubMed (Index Medicus),* MEDLINE/MEDLARS, SciSearch, Research Alert, and Neuroscience Citation Index.

PROGRAM OBJECTIVE
The goal of *Neuroimaging Clinics of North America* is to keep practicing radiologists and radiology residents up to date with current clinical practice in radiology by providing timely articles reviewing the state of the art in patient care.

TARGET AUDIENCE
Practicing radiologists, radiology residents, and other healthcare professionals who utilize neuroimaging findings to provide patient care.

LEARNING OBJECTIVES
Upon completion of this activity, participants will be able to:
1. Review current thyroid cancer guidelines and treatments as well as future prospects of imaging modalities.
2. Discuss differentiation and diagnosis of common benign and malignant diseases affecting the thyroid gland.
3. Recognize the impact preoperative imaging of lymph nodes has on surgical decision making and patient outcomes.

ACCREDITATION
The Elsevier Office of Continuing Medical Education (EOCME) is accredited by the Accreditation Council for Continuing Medical Education (ACCME) to provide continuing medical education for physicians.

The EOCME designates this journal-based CME activity for a maximum of 11 *AMA PRA Category 1 Credit*(s)™. Physicians should claim only the credit commensurate with the extent of their participation in the activity.

All other healthcare professionals requesting continuing education credit for this enduring material will be issued a certificate of participation.

DISCLOSURE OF CONFLICTS OF INTEREST
The EOCME assesses conflict of interest with its instructors, faculty, planners, and other individuals who are in a position to control the content of CME activities. All relevant conflicts of interest that are identified are thoroughly vetted by EOCME for fair balance, scientific objectivity, and patient care recommendations. EOCME is committed to providing its learners with CME activities that promote improvements or quality in healthcare and not a specific proprietary business or a commercial interest.

The planning committee, staff, authors and editors listed below have identified no financial relationships or relationships to products or devices they or their spouse/life partner have with commercial interest related to the content of this CME activity:
Salmaan Ahmed, MD; Diana Bell, MD; Maria E. Cabanillas, MD; Susana Calle, MD; Noah Nathan Chasen, MD; Regina Chavous-Gibson, MSN, RN; Jeanie Choi, MD; Uriel Clemente-Gutierrez, MD; James Matthew Debnam, MD; Bita Esmaeli, MD; Qiong Gan, MD; Edward G. Grant, MD; Xu Guofan, MD; Kirthi Koka, MS; Pradeep Kuttysankaran; Kim O. Learned, MD; Harshawn S. Malhi, MD; Suresh K. Mukherji, MD, MBA, FACR; Kylan Naidoo; Nancy D. Perrier, MD; C. Douglas Phillips, MD; Eric Rohren, MD, PhD; Michelle Roytman, MD; Komal Shah, MD; Aditya S. Shirali, MD; Sara B. Strauss, MD; Devaki Shilpa Sudha Surasi, MD; Jeena Varghese, MD; John Vassallo; Daniel Vinh, MD; Jennifer Rui Wang, MD, ScM; Michelle D. Williams, MD; Divya Yadav, MD; Mark Zafereo, MD.

UNAPPROVED/OFF-LABEL USE DISCLOSURE
The EOCME requires CME faculty to disclose to the participants:
1. When products or procedures being discussed are off-label, unlabelled, experimental, and/or investigational (not US Food and Drug Administration [FDA] approved); and
2. Any limitations on the information presented, such as data that are preliminary or that represent ongoing research, interim analyses, and/or unsupported opinions. Faculty may discuss information about pharmaceutical agents that is outside of FDA-approved labelling. This information is intended solely for CME and is not intended to promote off-label use of these medications. If you have any questions, contact the medical affairs department of the manufacturer for the most recent prescribing information.

TO ENROLL
To enroll in the *Neuroimaging Clinics of North America* Continuing Medical Education program, call customer service at 1-800-654-2452 or sign up online at http://www.theclinics.com/home/cme. The CME program is available to subscribers for an additional annual fee of USD 265.00.

METHOD OF PARTICIPATION
In order to claim credit, participants must complete the following:
1. Complete enrolment as indicated above.
2. Read the activity.
3. Complete the CME Test and Evaluation. Participants must achieve a score of 70% on the test. All CME Tests and Evaluations must be completed online.

CME INQUIRIES/SPECIAL NEEDS
For all CME inquiries or special needs, please contact elsevierCME@elsevier.com.

NEUROIMAGING CLINICS OF NORTH AMERICA

SERIES OF RELATED INTEREST

Advances in Clinical Radiology
Available at: Advancesinclinicalradiology.com
MRI Clinics of North America
Available at: MRI.theclinics.com
PET Clinics
Available at: https://www.pet.theclinics.com/
Radiologic Clinics of North America
Available at: Radiologic.theclinics.com

THE CLINICS ARE AVAILABLE ONLINE!
Access your subscription at:
www.theclinics.com

Contributors

CONSULTING EDITOR

SURESH K. MUKHERJI, MD, MBA, FACR
Clinical Professor, Marian University, Director of Head and Neck Radiology, ProScan Imaging, Regional Medical Director, Envision Physician Services, Carmel, Indiana, USA

EDITORS

SALMAAN AHMED, MD
Associate Professor, Division of Diagnostic Imaging, Department of Neuroradiology, The University of Texas MD Anderson Cancer Center, Houston, Texas, USA

JAMES MATTHEW DEBNAM, MD
Professor, Division of Diagnostic Imaging, Department of Neuroradiology, The University of Texas MD Anderson Cancer Center, Houston, Texas, USA

AUTHORS

SALMAAN AHMED, MD
Associate Professor, Division of Diagnostic Imaging, Department of Neuroradiology, The University of Texas MD Anderson Cancer Center, Houston, Texas, USA

DIANA BELL, MD
Associate Professor, Head and Neck Section, Departments of Pathology and Head and Neck Surgery, The University of Texas MD Anderson Cancer Center, Houston, Texas, USA

MARIA E. CABANILLAS, MD
Departments of Endocrine Neoplasia and Hormonal Disorders, The University of Texas MD Anderson Cancer Center, Houston, Texas, USA

SUSANA CALLE, MD
Assistant Professor, Department of Neuroradiology, Division of Diagnostic Imaging, The University of Texas MD Anderson Cancer Center, Houston, Texas, USA

NOAH NATHAN CHASEN, MD
Assistant Professor, Department of Neuroradiology, The University of Texas MD Anderson Cancer Center, Houston, Texas, USA

JEANIE CHOI, MD
Associate Professor, Neuroradiology Section, Department of Diagnostic and Interventional Imaging, The University of Texas Health Science Center at Houston, Houston, Texas, USA

URIEL CLEMENTE-GUTIERREZ, MD
Postdoctoral Research Fellow, Section of Surgical Endocrinology, Department of Surgical Oncology, The University of Texas MD Anderson Cancer Center, Houston, Texas, USA

JAMES MATTHEW DEBNAM, MD
Professor, Division of Diagnostic Imaging, Department of Neuroradiology, The University of Texas MD Anderson Cancer Center, Houston, Texas, USA

BITA ESMAELI, MD
Ophthalmic Plastic Surgery, The University of Texas MD Anderson Cancer Center, Houston, Texas, USA

QIONG GAN, MD
Assistant Professor, Department of Anatomical Pathology, The University of Texas MD Anderson Cancer Center, Houston, Texas, USA

EDWARD G. GRANT, MD
Professor of Radiology, University of Southern California, Keck USC Hospital, Los Angeles, California, USA

XU GUOFAN, MD
Assistant Professor, Department of Nuclear Medicine, The University of Texas MD Anderson Cancer Center, Houston, Texas, USA

KIRTHI KOKA, MS
Ophthalmic Plastic Surgery, The University of Texas MD Anderson Cancer Center, Houston, Texas, USA; Orbit, Oculoplasty, Reconstructive and Aesthetic Services, Sankara Nethralaya, Chennai, India

KIM O. LEARNED, MD
Associate Professor, Department of Neuroradiology, Division of Diagnostic Imaging, The University of Texas MD Anderson Cancer Center, Houston, Texas, USA

HARSHAWN S. MALHI, MD
Associate Professor, Department of Radiology, Keck School of Medicine of USC, University of Southern California, Los Angeles, California, USA

KYLAN NAIDOO
Department of Abdominal Imaging, Summer Student Program, Division of Diagnostic Imaging, The University of Texas MD Anderson Cancer Center, Houston, Texas, USA

NANCY D. PERRIER, MD
Chief, Section of Surgical Endocrinology, Department of Surgical Oncology, Associate Director of Endocrine Center, The University of Texas MD Anderson Cancer Center, Houston, Texas, USA

C. DOUGLAS PHILLIPS, MD
Professor of Radiology, Department of Radiology, Weill Cornell Medical College, NewYork-Presbyterian Hospital, New York, New York, USA

ERIC ROHREN, MD, PhD
Professor and Chair, Department of Radiology, Baylor College of Medicine, Houston, Texas, USA

MICHELLE ROYTMAN, MD
Neuroradiology Fellow, Department of Radiology, Weill Cornell Medical College,

NewYork-Presbyterian Hospital, New York, New York, USA

KOMAL SHAH, MD
Department of Neuroradiology, Division of Diagnostic Imaging, The University of Texas MD Anderson Cancer Center, Houston, Texas, USA

ADITYA S. SHIRALI, MD
Surgical Endocrinology Fellow, Section of Surgical Endocrinology, Department of Surgical Oncology, The University of Texas MD Anderson Cancer Center, Houston, Texas, USA

SARA B. STRAUSS, MD
Assistant Professor of Radiology, Department of Radiology, Weill Cornell Medical College, NewYork-Presbyterian Hospital, New York, New York, USA

DEVAKI SHILPA SUDHA SURASI, MD
Department of Nuclear Medicine, Division of Diagnostic Imaging, The University of Texas MD Anderson Cancer Center, Houston, Texas, USA

JEENA VARGHESE, MD
Assistant Professor, Endocrine Neoplasia and Hormonal Disorders, The University of Texas MD Anderson Cancer Center, Houston, Texas, USA

DANIEL VINH, MD
Department of Otolaryngology - Head and Neck Surgery, Baylor College of Medicine, Houston, Texas, USA

JENNIFER RUI WANG, MD, ScM
Assistant Professor, Department of Head and Neck Surgery, The University of Texas MD Anderson Cancer Center, Houston, Texas, USA

MICHELLE D. WILLIAMS, MD
Professor, Department of Pathology, Chief, Head and Neck Section, The University of Texas MD Anderson Cancer Center, Houston, Texas, USA

DIVYA YADAV, MD
Post-doctoral fellow, Department of Radiation Oncology, The University of Texas MD Anderson Cancer Center, Houston, Texas, USA

MARK ZAFEREO, MD
Department of Otolaryngology - Head and Neck Surgery, The University of Texas MD Anderson Cancer Center, Houston, Texas, USA

Contents

> Imaging evaluation of the thyroid gland spans a plethora of modalities, including ultra-sound imaging, cross-sectional studies, and nuclear medicine techniques. The overlapping of clinical and imaging findings of benign and malignant thyroid disease can make interpretation a complex undertaking. We aim to review and simplify the vast current literature and provide a practical approach to the imaging of thyroid disease for application in daily practice. Our approach highlights the keys to differentiating and diagnosing common benign and malignant disease affecting the thyroid gland.

> Benign or malignant thyroid nodules are common in adults. Fine needle aspiration biopsy is the gold standard for diagnosis. Most thyroid nodules are benign. Ultra-sound imaging is the optimal noninvasive imaging modality to determine which nodules demonstrate malignant features. The American College of Radiology Thyroid Imaging Reporting and Data System committee published a standardized approach to classifying nodules on ultrasound. The ultrasound features in this system are categorized as benign, minimally suspicious, moderately suspicious, or highly suspicious for malignancy. Applying the Thyroid Imaging Reporting and Data System results in a meaningful decrease in the number of thyroid nodules biopsied.

> Robust molecular testing is commercially available for adjuvant assessment of cytologically indeterminate thyroid nodules. Testing has been developed and optimized for fine needle aspiration biopsy collections of thyroid nodules typically under ultra-sound evaluation. These assays use a combination of gene expression and/or DNA and RNA assessments for molecular alterations to stratify indeterminate thyroid nodules as benign with risk level similar to benign cytologic read or suspicious with increased risk of malignancy. Guidelines for when to consider adjuvant molecular testing will be discussed.

> Sonographic evaluation of cervical lymph nodes in patients with thyroid malignancy is important both for preoperative staging and for post-treatment surveillance, and

contrast-enhanced computed tomography plays a complementary role. Knowledge of anatomy and surgical approaches, combined with an understanding of the various imaging features that distinguish malignant from benign lymph nodes, allows for accurate staging, thereby enabling complete surgical initial resection.

Management of thyroid cancer requires a multidisciplinary approach including head and neck/endocrine surgeons, endocrinologists, oncologists, and radiologists. The radiographic evaluation of thyroid cancer is critical for complete and precise staging and affects the surgical approach to address these cancers. The purpose of this article is to briefly review the common thyroid cancer pathologies and surgical considerations in thyroid cancer, focusing on the extent of surgery and the influence of preoperative imaging on surgical decision-making. This article assumes that a diagnosis of thyroid cancer has been made and does not discuss the workup or surveillance of thyroid nodules.

Thyroid hormones T3 and T4 are crucial for development and differentiation of various cells in the body. They are also essential for regulating metabolism in nearly all tissues. Iodine is an integral element in the synthesis of thyroid hormone and is actively transported into the thyroid by a Na^+ /I^- symporter. The thyroid can take up radioactive iodine just like it would take iodine and hence can be used to evaluate and treat several thyroid diseases. Radioactive iodine is one of the first radioisotopes to be used in medicine.

Primary thyroid cancers demonstrate distinct biological behaviors depending on their histologic characteristics. The ability to accumulate radioiodine by differentiated thyroid cancer cells is lost in primary aggressive, poorly differentiated and dedifferentiated tumor cells. PET imaging comes into play in these challenging situations where it can provide additive information to radioiodine scintigraphy and conventional imaging. This review focuses on the current guidelines and future prospects of PET imaging in thyroid cancers.

Differentiated and anaplastic thyroid cancer are tumors derived from follicular thyroid cancers and are clinically and genetically distinct. Treatment of these tumors has evolved over the past decade, with 6 drugs/drug combinations that are US Food and Drug Administration approved.

Graves disease is an autoimmune disorder caused by the breakdown of immune tolerance to thyroid antigens against the TSH receptor. In approximately 25% of patients, an inflammatory condition, Graves eye disease (GED), affects the orbital soft tissues. About 60% of patients develop mild symptoms including fat expansion and inflammation of the levator muscle complex with resultant proptosis, eyelid retraction, and exposure of the globe. The remaining patients experience enlargement of one or more of the extraocular muscles, conjunctival and eyelid edema and congestion, restricted ocular movement with resultant diplopia, and optic nerve compression leading to compressive optic neuropathy.

Primary hyperparathyroidism results most commonly from a parathyroid adenoma, a benign parathyroid tumor that causes high levels of parathyroid hormone production. Given recent advances in surgical techniques allowing more focused, minimally invasive procedures, presurgical identification of candidate operative tissue has become increasingly useful in avoidance of 4-gland exploration. Imaging modalities for identification of parathyroid adenoma include ultrasonography, parathyroid scintigraphy, four-dimensional computed tomography, and magnetic resonance imaging. This article discusses technical and interpretive approaches for the available modalities, and reviews their strengths and weaknesses. Updates to the individual modalities and approaches for problem solving in lesion detection are also addressed.

Surgical intervention remains the mainstay of treatment of hyperparathyroidism and provides the highest chance at cure. After the disease is confirmed by biochemical testing, surgeons must use a combination of patient clinical history and radiographic imaging to determine the most appropriate surgical strategy. Through either minimally invasive parathyroidectomy or bilateral cervical exploration, surgeons provide high rates of cure for hyperparathyroidism with low rates of persistence or recurrence.

Foreword
Thyroid and Parathyroid Imaging

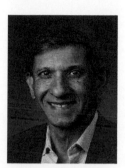

Suresh K. Mukherji, MD, MBA, FACR
Consulting Editor

Thyroid disorders have always been one of the most challenging areas for me. Thyroid imaging is "shared" by many radiologists, including the subspecialists (neuroradiologists, nuclear medicine, and so forth) and modality (ultrasound, PET/CT). As a Head & Neck/Neuroradiologist, I have always had a hard time keeping abreast of the latest advances in thyroid and parathyroid diseases because the advances have occurred in multiple disciplines.

Fortunately, this issue provides a comprehensive evidenced-based update on the state-of-the-art diagnosis and management of thyroid and parathyroid pathologic condition. There are articles devoted to a variety of thyroid and parathyroid disorders with specific articles focused on the diagnosis, staging, management, and treatment of thyroid carcinoma.

I would like to personally thank Drs Salmaan Ahmed and Matthew Debnam for coediting this wonderful issue. This issue is truly multidisciplinary with articles authored by internationally renowned experts who have contributed directly to the advances made within the past decade toward managing thyroid and parathyroid diseases. I am both honored and grateful to the editors and authors for their outstanding contributions!

Suresh K. Mukherji, MD, MBA, FACR
Clinical Professor, Marian University
Director of Head & Neck Radiology
ProScan Imaging, Regional Medical Director
Envision Physician Services Carmel, Indiana, USA

E-mail address:
sureshmukherji@hotmail.com

https://doi.org/10.1016/j.nic.2021.05.002
1052-5149/21/

Foreword

Thyroid and Parathyroid Imaging

Suresh K. Mukherji, MD, MBA, FACR
Consulting Editor

Thyroid disorders have always been one of the most challenging areas for me. Thyroid imaging is "shared" by many radiologists, including the subspecialists (neuroradiologists, nuclear medicine, and so forth) and modality (ultrasound, PET/CT). As a Head & Neck/Neuroradiologist, I have always had a hard time keeping abreast of the latest advances in thyroid and parathyroid diseases, because the advances have occurred in multiple disciplines.

Fortunately, this issue provides a comprehensive evidence-based update on the state-of-the-art diagnosis and management of thyroid and parathyroid pathologic condition. There are articles devoted to a variety of thyroid and parathyroid disorders with specific articles focused on the diagnosis, staging, management, and treatment of thyroid carcinoma.

I would like to personally thank Drs Salmaan Ahmad and Matthew Debnam for coediting this wonderful issue. This issue is truly multidisciplinary with articles authored by internationally renowned experts who have contributed directly to the advances made within the past decade toward managing thyroid and parathyroid diseases. I am both honored and grateful to the editors and authors for their outstanding contributions!

Suresh K. Mukherji, MD, MBA, FACR
Clinical Professor, Marian University
Director of Head & Neck Radiology
ProScan Imaging, Regional Medical Director
Envision Physician Services Carmel, Indiana, USA

E-mail address:
sureshmukherji@hotmail.com

Neuroimag Clin N Am 31 (2021) xi
https://doi.org/10.1016/j.nic.2021.05.003
1052-5149/21/© 2021 Elsevier Inc. All rights reserved.

Preface
Thyroid and Parathyroid Imaging

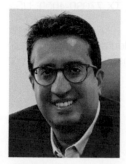 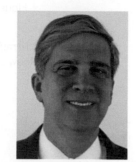

Salmaan Ahmed, MD   James Matthew Debnam, MD
Editors

Over the past decade, there has been a significant increase in the diagnosis of thyroid cancer coupled with advances in the triage of thyroid nodules and management of thyroid cancer. In particular, the development of the Thyroid Imaging Reporting and Data System (TIRADS) allows for an evidenced-based standardized approach to reduce the number of ultrasound-guided fine needle aspirations (FNAs) performed on benign nodules and the majority of the small well-differentiated thyroid cancers that may not meet size criteria for biopsy, as these are likely indolent.

Preoperative molecular testing of the FNA sample has emerged as a useful adjunct to the cytological evaluation and is now widely used to predict the risk of malignancy within nodules that are not definitively benign or malignant on initial cytologic assessment. Nodules with a low likelihood of malignancy based on molecular testing can now be triaged to observation, thereby sparing these patients a potential thyroid lobectomy.

Remarkable strides have been made in the management of anaplastic thyroid carcinoma (ATC) over the past 5 years, with significant improvements in survival of patients treated at our institution.

At MD Anderson Cancer Center (MDACC), patients with thyroid and parathyroid pathologic condition are evaluated in a dedicated neck ultrasound clinic that was established in 2005 within the Department of Neuroradiology. Case volumes of approximately 6800 cases in 2007 have now more than doubled to greater than 16,000 in 2018. At present, there are 9 examination rooms dedicated entirely to neck ultrasound with 9 full-time sonographers and 3 medical assistants. Patients requiring FNA or core biopsy can have the procedure performed concurrently with the diagnostic ultrasound exam. An onsite attending cytologist provides preliminary cytologic results that are typically available within 20 minutes following completion of FNA. Patients then typically proceed to a same-day clinic visit with the endocrinologist and/or surgeon.

While sonography of the neck soft tissues and thyroid is typically performed by general radiologists and body imagers worldwide, our existing MDACC neck ultrasound clinic reflects the preferences of our endocrinologists and surgeons to optimize patient outcomes.

In this issue of the *Neuroimaging Clinics*, we provide a comprehensive evidenced-based update on the state-of-the-art diagnosis and the management of thyroid and parathyroid pathologic condition. We are fortunate to have the articles in this issue written by internationally renowned experts, who have contributed directly to the advances made within the past decade toward managing thyroid and parathyroid diseases.

Dr. Debnam and I are grateful for this opportunity to contribute to the literature and thank Dr. Suresh Mukherji as well as Karen Solomon and John Vassallo at Elsevier for the ongoing support. We acknowledge the outstanding team of sonographers, neuroradiologists, surgeons, endocrinologist, and pathologists at MDACC, many of whom are authors on this project.

Neuroimag Clin N Am 31 (2021) xiii–xiv
https://doi.org/10.1016/j.nic.2021.05.001

Dedication:
Dr. Ahmed: To my daughters Mischa (8) and Sophia (5), for the immense joy and fulfillment they bring to my life.
Dr. Debnam: To my wife Stacy, and our children Celeste and Andrew.

Salmaan Ahmed, MD
Division of Diagnostic Imaging
Department of Neuroradiology
UT
MD Anderson Cancer Center
1400 Pressler Street, Unit 1482
Houston, TX 77030, USA

James Matthew Debnam, MD
Division of Diagnostic Imaging
Department of Neuroradiology
UT
MD Anderson Cancer Center
1515 Holcombe Boulevard, Unit 1482
Houston, TX 77030-4009, USA

E-mail addresses:
Salmaan.Ahmed@mdanderson.org (S. Ahmed)
matthew.debnam@mdanderson.org
(J.M. Debnam)

Imaging of the Thyroid
Practical Approach

Susana Calle, MD[a],*, Jeanie Choi, MD[b], Salmaan Ahmed, MD[a], Diana Bell, MD[c],
Kim O. Learned, MD[a]

KEYWORDS

• Thyroid • Imaging • Benign • Malignant • Cross-sectional • Ultrasound

KEY POINTS

- Ultrasound examination is a cost-effective modality for diagnostic purposes and biopsy guidance in thyroid disease. Computed tomography is the workhorse for thyroid tumor staging. Radionuclide scintigraphy evaluates thyroid function.
- Thyroid imaging features can be classified as either diffuse or focal.
- Diffuse multinodular goiter and thyroiditis are common benign conditions. Focal nodules should be evaluated sonographically for benign and malignant features using Thyroid Imaging and Data System guidelines.
- Imaging detection of local invasiveness of a thyroid lesion and nodal metastasis may lead to expedient diagnosis of aggressive thyroid malignancy.
- Key imaging features suspicious for malignancy in a background of diffuse benign disease include focal highly suspicious hypoechoic nodule, microcalcifications, asymmetric lobar involvement and focal fluoro-2-deoxy-D-glucose avidity.

INTRODUCTION

The thyroid gland plays a critical role in regulating metabolic functions and imaging has long been established as an essential element in the workup of abnormal thyroid function and clinically suspected lesions of the thyroid gland. Knowledge of the imaging modalities as well as normal and abnormal imaging appearances of the thyroid gland and pathologies is essential for appropriate identification and diagnosis of thyroid lesions. In this article, we discuss the pertinent anatomy and nodal drainage and review the imaging appearance of common thyroid diseases, with a special emphasis on a practical imaging approach to expedient diagnosis of highly prevalent thyroid conditions such as Grave's disease, goiter,

thyroiditis, and thyroid cancer. The relative roles of various imaging modalities in the evaluation of various thyroid diseases are included.

ANATOMY

The thyroid gland is a shield-shaped gland located superficially in the infrahyoid neck over the cricoid and trachea (**Fig. 1**). The right and left thyroid lobe join inferiorly by a thin band of tissue over the anterior trachea known as the isthmus. Anteriorly, the thyroid gland abuts the strap musculature and sternocleidomastoid muscles. The carotid arteries and jugular veins are located lateral and posterior to the gland, and the posterior margin of the thyroid abuts the longus coli muscles.[1] An accessory, pyramidal lobe, is present in approximately 50% to

---

The authors have no pertinent commercial or financial conflicts of interest to disclose.
[a] Department of Neuroradiology, Division of Diagnostic Imaging, The University of Texas MD Anderson Cancer Center, 1400 Pressler Street Unit 1482, Houston, TX 77030, USA; [b] Neuroradiology Section, Department of Diagnostic and Interventional Imaging, The University of Texas Health Science Center at Houston, 6431 Fannin Street, Houston, TX 77030, USA; [c] Head and Neck Section, Departments of Pathology and Head and Neck Surgery, The University of Texas MD Anderson Cancer Center, 1515 Holcombe Boulevard, Houston, TX 77030, USA
* Corresponding author.
E-mail address: susanacalle@gmail.com

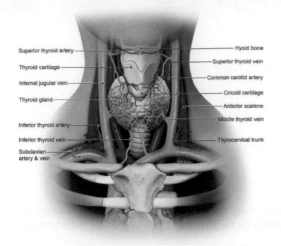

Fig. 1. Illustration of the thyroid gland and anatomic landmarks. (*Courtesy of* Kelly Kage, MFA, CMI, Houston, TX.)

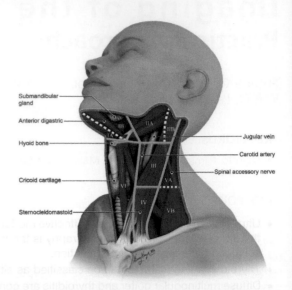

Fig. 2. Illustration of the nodal compartments of the neck. (*Courtesy of* Kelly Kage, MFA, CMI, Houston, TX.)

70% of the population and arises from the isthmus and extends superiorly along the course of the distal thyroglossal duct.[2]

A thin fibrous capsule surrounds the thyroid gland with septated projections that extend into the thyroid parenchyma to divide thyroid tissue into lobules. A rich vascular network is supplied by paired superior and inferior thyroidal arteries, which are branches of the external carotid arteries and thyrocervical trunks, respectively. The thyroid gland receives innervation from the vagus nerve and the cervical sympathetic plexus, which influence gland perfusion.[2]

Lymphatic drainage of the gland includes the deep lateral cervical nodal levels I to V, the central anterior nodal levels VI to VII (prelaryngeal/Delphian, pretracheal, paratracheal, and superior mediastinum) and retropharyngeal nodal groups. Although the inferior portions of the gland and the isthmus tend to drain to the paratracheal and lower deep cervical level III to IV nodes, the superior gland drains into the superior pretracheal, prelaryngeal/Delphian, and level II to III cervical groups, explaining the propensity of skip metastasis to the upper nodal group in tumors arising from the upper pole of the thyroid.[3]

For the specific purpose of multidisciplinary agreement in staging and management of thyroid carcinoma, the American Joint Committee on Cancer and the American Thyroid Association (ATA) use the classic I to VI cervical nodal stations to describe pertinent nodal disease[4,5] (Fig. 2). The benefits of the nodal classification method are reproducible consistency mapping with the limits of the compartments readily identified on imaging, clear surgical correlates, and consensus

communication across specialties. Thyroid cancer nodal staging is defined by central anterior compartment (level VI and VII), or lateral compartment (levels I–V) and retropharyngeal nodal metastasis, and is detailed in an article in this series, titled Imaging of Cervical Lymph Nodes in Thyroid Cancer: Ultrasound and Computed Tomography by Chasen and colleagues.

IMAGING FINDINGS
Ultrasound Imaging

Ultrasound examination constitutes the most sensitive imaging modality in the evaluation of the thyroid gland. Added benefits include availability, low cost, and lack of ionizing radiation.[1] Real-time ultrasound examination performed with high-resolution linear array transducers ranging from 7.5 to 12.0 MHz provides detailed evaluation of focal and diffuse thyroid disease and assessment of cervical nodes. Additionally, ultrasound examination is essential in guiding fine-needle aspiration procedures for histopathologic diagnosis.

The normal appearance of the thyroid gland on ultrasound examination is that of a well-defined homogeneous gland, which is hyperechoic relative to adjacent musculature and is draped along the anterior trachea.[1] On average, the thyroid isthmus measures 3 mm in thickness and each lobe measures 4 to 6 cm in length and up to 2 cm in both transverse and anteroposterior dimensions.[1]

Cross-sectional Imaging

Cross-sectional imaging modalities, including computed tomography (CT) scans and MR imaging of the neck, are an important adjunct in the evaluation of patients with thyroid disease, and obtained from the level of the tracheal bifurcation inferiorly to the skull base superiorly. These techniques allow for the interrogation of disease extent and nodal stations not readily accessible to ultrasound examination, including the lateral retropharyngeal compartments and retrosternal upper mediastinum. Furthermore, cross-sectional imaging allows for the characterization of tumor invasion into deep and neighboring structures, which upstages thyroid malignancies.[2] Gross extrathyroidal extension (ETE) to the strap muscles will upstage to T3b disease, regardless of tumor size for thyroid cancer.[5] The invasion of tissue beyond the strap muscles, including subcutaneous soft tissues, larynx, trachea, esophagus, and recurrent laryngeal nerve, would classify the primary tumor as T4a and extension to the prevertebral fascia or encasement of carotid or mediastinal vessels as T4b.[5] The commonly encountered thyroid cancers and discussion of changes in staging in the most recent American Joint Committee on Cancer, eighth edition, will be highlighted in malignant thyroid disease section elsewhere int his article.

On CT imaging, owing to the iodine content of the thyroid, the gland is intrinsically hyperdense on noncontrast imaging with Hounsfield units ranging from 80 to 100. Iodinated contrast administration is recommended for better evaluation of the gland, which shows avid homogenous enhancement, the surrounding structures, and cervical nodes.[6] Iodine is generally cleared within 4 to 8 weeks in most patients, so concern about iodine burden from intravenous contrast causing a clinically significant delay in subsequent whole-body radioactive iodine scan or radioactive iodine ablation treatment after the contrast CT imaging followed by surgery is generally unfounded.[4]

MR imaging allows for improved soft tissue differentiation, whereas CT scans have greater spatial resolution and remains the imaging workhorse.[7] The neck MR imaging generally includes a T1-weighted image, T2-weighted sequence, fat-saturated T2-weighted sequence, followed by postcontrast fat-saturated T1-weighted images. The normal appearance of the thyroid gland is that of a homogeneous, smoothly marginated parenchyma that is, isointense on T1, slightly hyperintense on T2, and demonstrates homogeneous enhancement compared with adjacent muscle.[7]

The soft tissue differentiation provided by MR imaging allows for the characterization of diffuse and focal thyroid disease. Findings of diffuse thyroid disease include variations in size, signal intensity, enhancement degree and pattern, and margin contour.[7] Furthermore, studies have explored the diagnostic potentials of MR imaging, including diffusion-weighted imaging, T2 signal intensity, and dynamic contrast-enhanced parameters, for the characterization of benign and malignant thyroid nodules.[8] In 1 study, the T2 signal intensity ratio is calculated by measuring the mean signal intensity of the nodule divided by the signal intensity of the paraspinal muscle, and both the T2 signal intensity ratio and the apparent diffusion coefficient values in papillary thyroid carcinoma (PTC) were significantly lower than for benign nodules.[8–10] These studies offer promising results in the classification of thyroid nodules, but the heterogeneity of diffusion and perfusion techniques, time consuming and cumbersome postprocessing, and higher cost hinder their widespread application and validation at this time.

Nuclear Medicine

Radionuclide imaging has been available for many years and allows for excellent functional evaluation of the thyroid gland. The most frequently used radiotracers in thyroid scintigraphy include technetium-99m pertechnetate and iodine-based tracers, including ^{123}I and [131]I. Additionally, gallium-67 may be used in the evaluation of thyroid lymphoma.

Scintigraphic imaging with I[123] is valuable in the characterization of thyroid nodules as either "hot" or "cold," depending on whether there is focal radiotracer accumulation or a focal photopenic defect, respectively.[11] Cold thyroid nodules have a greater incidence of malignancy, calculated at 10% to 20%, and therefore require further evaluation with possible biopsy. Conversely, hot nodules in the setting of low thyroid-stimulating hormone, are generally benign and may not require further studies.[11] [131]I is beneficial in the acquisition of whole body imaging following thyroidectomy and thyroid ablation for the detection of residual tissue and metastatic disease.[11]

The normal thyroid gland on PET imaging using 2-[fluorine-18] fluoro-2-deoxy-D-glucose (FDG) shows homogeneous radiotracer uptake similar to that of adjacent muscle.[11] PET-CT scanning relies on high glucose metabolism and therefore increased tracer uptake will generally be greater in cases of poor tumor differentiation with a greater risk of metastatic disease. For this reason, PET is generally used in high-risk patients and is not routinely recommended for determining disease extent in low-risk populations.[12]

It has been estimated that approximately 2% to 3% of PET imaging reveals an incidental thyroid nodule. Although higher standardized uptake value measurements have been documented in malignant versus in benign nodules, no specific threshold has been defined to predict malignancy. However, increased uptake has been associated with a 14% to 40% greater increase in risk of malignancy and should therefore prompt further evaluation with ultrasound examination and ultrasound-guided biopsy if pertinent.[11] The management of FDG-avid nodules on PET/CT is further addressed in the article of this series, titled PET/Computed Tomography in Thyroid Cancer by Yadav and colleagues.

PRACTICAL APPROACH TO IMAGING EVALUATION

When confronted with thyroid disorders, it is beneficial to establish a basic mental framework that will allow the radiologist to categorize the entity in a broad fashion (Fig. 3). First, imaging features of the thyroid gland can be classified as either diffuse or focal. Diffuse abnormality of the thyroid gland must prompt the radiologist to consider multinodular goiter and the spectrum of thyroiditis, which are generally benign conditions. However, it is important to recognize instances where diffuse infiltration of the gland may signify malignant pathology, such as with the diffuse sclerosing variant of PTC, and keen attention to detect malignancy within the diffuse benign disease, such as the development of PTC and/or lymphoma in the setting of Hashimoto thyroiditis and diffuse metastatic infiltration of the thyroid gland.

Conversely, focal lesions and each nodule in the multinodular goiter should be evaluated for benign or malignant features to determine management.

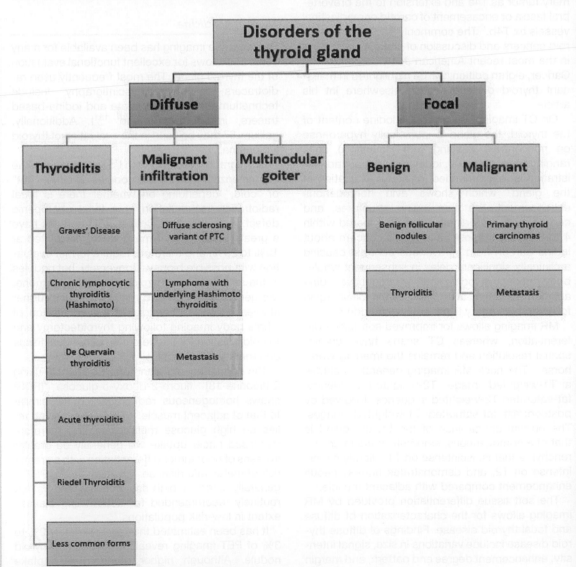

Fig. 3. General approach to classification of disorders of the thyroid gland.

The implementation of the Thyroid Imaging and Data System (TI-RADS) and ATA guidelines aid in determining the risk of malignancy and the subsequent management strategies for thyroid nodules based on imaging features pertaining to nodule composition, echotexture, and shape, among other features. The assessment and classification of thyroid nodules will be addressed in detail in the article of this series, titled Ultrasound of Thyroid Nodules and the Thyroid Imaging Reporting and Data System by Harshawn Malhi and Edward Grant.

The thorough exploration of cervical nodes serves as an important adjunct in the diagnosis of thyroid pathology. The presence of unilateral versus bilateral adenopathy has different implications as does size, echogenicity, morphology, and vascularity. Normal and reactive nodes tend to be oval shaped and slightly hypoechoic to muscle with central echogenic hila and organized flow on Doppler imaging.[13] In contrast, thyroid nodal metastases will display cystic transformation, internal calcifications, or hyperechogenic foci with 100% specificity and positive predictive value as well as less specific suspicious findings of rounded morphology and disorganized vascular flow.[13,14] The article of this series, titled Imaging of Cervical Lymph Nodes in Thyroid Cancer: Ultrasound and Computed Tomography by Chasen and colleagues, goes into greater detail regarding benign and malignant nodal imaging features.

Furthermore, attention to key points pertaining to clinical presentation may also help narrow down differential considerations further. For instance, a nontender goiter and hypothyroidism in the setting of diffuse thyroid infiltration may alert to Hashimoto thyroiditis. Conversely, a painful transient thyrotoxic state with suppressed thyroid-stimulating hormone can indicate subacute thyroiditis.[15] Similarly, a rapidly progressing thyroid mass with imaging signs of ETE should raise suspicion for anaplastic thyroid carcinoma. These clues pertaining to the patient's symptomatology, among others, are essential in guiding diagnosis and therapy.

BENIGN THYROID DISEASE
Graves' Disease

Graves' disease is an autoimmune condition wherein autoantibodies are produced against thyroid proteins, most notably to the thyroid-stimulating hormone receptor.[16] The resultant effects include hyperplasia of the thyroid with accompanying autonomous function of the gland and hyperthyroidism with elevated free T3 and T4 levels in the setting of decreased serum thyroid-stimulating hormone. This entity is more common in females between the ages of 20 and 50 years.[16] The clinical presentation is characterized by a triad consisting of hypertrophy of the thyroid gland, exophthalmos secondary to infiltrative ophthalmopathy, and pretibial myxedema. Although the basis of diagnosis lies in the clinical and laboratory features of the disease, imaging with ultrasound and Doppler imaging of all hyperthyroid patients is generally widely recommended.[16,17]

Ultrasound features include diffuse enlargement of the gland, including the thyroid isthmus, with a rounded contour and variable echotexture. The gland may seem to be diffusely hypoechoic and heterogeneous or alternatively may be normal in echotexture. Exploration with Doppler imaging reveals a characteristically diffuse increase in parenchymal vascularity, termed "thyroid inferno" (Fig. 4). Of note, the degree of increased vascularity does not correlate directly with the level of hyperthyroidism and generally reflects inflammatory changes in the gland.[16]

Thyroid scintigraphy reveals diffuse enlargement of the gland with homogeneous elevation of radiotracer uptake at 24 hours relative to background activity owing to both increased function and increased stimulation.[18] The increased activity may result in the visualization of the pyramidal lobe that, owing to its small size, is not typically identified (see Fig. 4).[18]

Cross-sectional imaging with a CT scan and MR imaging is not generally recommended as a workup for presumptive Graves' disease. Findings are generally nonspecific revealing an enlarged gland with decreased Hounsfield units on CT imaging and avid enhancement and increase T1 and T2 signal intensity on MR imaging owing to parenchymal and vascularity changes.[19]

Thyroiditis

Thyroiditis, representing inflammation of the thyroid gland, generally manifests as diffuse heterogeneous echotexture on ultrasound with heterogeneous attenuation on CT imaging (Fig. 5). Exploration with Doppler imaging may additionally demonstrate widespread increased vascularity.[11] The entity can be subclassified as chronic lymphocytic thyroiditis, de Quervain thyroiditis, acute thyroiditis, Riedel thyroiditis, or other less common forms.[11] Chronic lymphocytic thyroiditis, also known as Hashimoto thyroiditis, is an autoimmune disorder and the most common cause of hypothyroidism in the United States. Histologically, this form of thyroiditis demonstrates a combination of inflammatory cells and Hurthle cells. Specifically, for Hashimoto thyroiditis to be diagnosed, specific

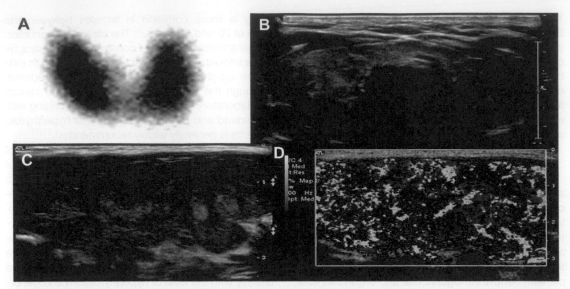

Fig. 4. Graves' disease. Thyroid scintigraphy (*A*) reveals diffuse thyroid enlargement with homogeneous increase in thyroid uptake at 24 hours. Transverse midline (*B*) and longitudinal view of the right thyroid lobe (*C*) grayscale ultrasound examination shows increased size of the thyroid gland, with rounded contours and heterogeneous echotexture. Exploration with color Doppler imaging (*D*) of the right thyroid lobe shows markedly increased parenchymal vascularity, termed "thyroid inferno."

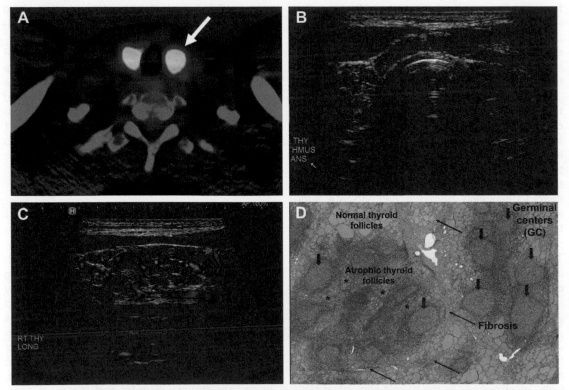

Fig. 5. Hashimoto thyroiditis. Axial fused FDG PET/CT image (*A*) shows diffusely increased FDG uptake with standardized uptake values of up to 12 (*white arrow*). Transverse midline (*B*) grayscale ultrasound imaging reveals heterogenous echotexture owing to a confluence of small hyperechoic nodules and micronodules with diffusely increased vascularity on power Doppler imaging (*C*). Histologic examination of tissue sample with hematoxylin and eosin staining (*D*) shows a combination of both normal and atrophic thyroid follicles, fibrosis and germinal centers.

antithyroid peroxidase and antithyroglobulin antibodies must be detected.

A common ultrasound appearance of Hashimoto thyroiditis is the heterogeneous echotexture of the thyroid parenchyma characterized by multiple hypoechoic micronodules (see **Fig. 5**). In Hashimoto thyroiditis, micronodulation corresponds to accentuated thyroid lobulation on the pathologic specimen. The reported positive predictive value for micronodulation in diagnosing Hashimoto thyroiditis was 94.7%. Sonographically, micronodules are generally 0.1 to 0.65 cm in size, hypoechoic, and surrounded by an echogenic rim. The hypoechogenicity of micronodules is due to massive infiltration by an exudate of lymphocytes and plasma cells similar to the hypoechogenicity caused by lymphoma. Formation of fibrous strands around the lobules causes a hyperechoic ring around each micronodule. The majority of micronodules, however, do not grow beyond 0.6 cm in size, distinguishing them from the larger hypoechoic lymphoma.[20] Ultrasound patterns associated with an 100% specificity for benignity include a "giraffe pattern" and the "white knight pattern," which are associated with Hashimoto thyroiditis.[21] The original giraffe pattern described by Bonavita is composed of thin hypoechoic septations surrounding rounded hyperechoic foci giving the lesion the appearance of giraffe fur (**Fig. 6**).[22] The white knight is a term given to a homogeneously hyperechoic nodule (**Fig. 7**). Correct identification of these patterns precludes the need for histologic confirmation.

The proposed association between Hashimoto thyroiditis and PTC remains a controversial topic. The frequent coexistence of these 2 entities suggests an underlying relationship. The prevalence of PTC in the setting of underlying Hashimoto thyroiditis is also greater than that in the general population. In patients who had undergone total thyroidectomy with a preoperative diagnosis of Hashimoto thyroiditis, the incidence of PTC was calculated at 40.2% for nodular variant Hashimoto thyroiditis and 8.1% for diffuse variant Hashimoto thyroiditis.[23] Conversely, in patients undergoing thyroidectomy for normofunctioning goiter, the incidence of PTC was reported at 7.7%.[23] The detection of focal hypoechoic nodule larger than the 0.6 cm size of micronodules in Hashimoto thyroiditis, clustered microcalcifications, or dystrophic calcification with asymmetric lobar involvement should prompt the radiologist to suspect PTC in the setting of underlying Hashimoto thyroiditis (**Fig. 8**). Furthermore, special attention must be paid to thorough assessment of cervical nodes for the detection of lateral cystic lymphadenopathy.

An additional association exists between Hashimoto thyroiditis and the development of primary thyroid lymphoma (PTL). Data suggesting their correlation include a greater reported incidence rate of PTL in patients with Hashimoto thyroiditis, reported at 16 persons per year per 10,000 persons, significantly higher than that of the general population, with some studies suggesting a 60-fold higher risk.[24] Furthermore, antithyroid peroxidase antibodies have been detected in approximately 60% to 80% of patients with PTL, which further indicates Hashimoto thyroiditis as a risk factor for the development of PTL.[24] It is suggested that the presence of lymphocytes in Hashimoto thyroiditis that undergo chronic antigenic stimulation predisposes them to malignant transformation.[24] On ultrasound examination, diffuse asymmetric enlargement of

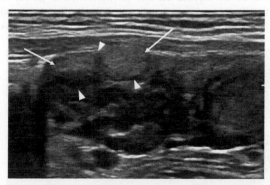

Fig. 6. Hashimoto thyroiditis. Longitudinal grayscale ultrasound of the thyroid parenchyma demonstrates a focal area with a giraffe pattern characterized by hyperechoic nodules (*arrows*) separated by hypoechoic septations (*arrowhead*).

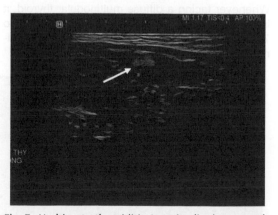

Fig. 7. Hashimoto thyroiditis. Longitudinal gray -scale ultrasound image of the right thyroid lobe shows homogeneously hyperechoic nodule termed the white knight (*arrow*) on a background of a diffusely heterogeneous parenchymal echotexture.

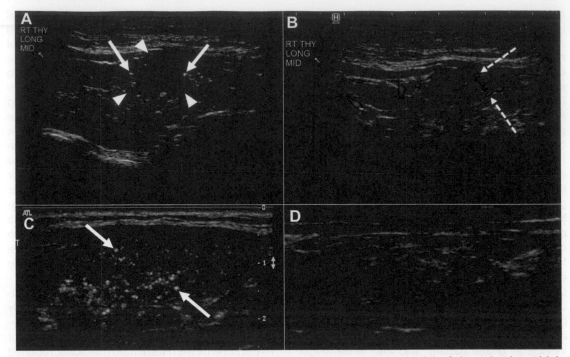

Fig. 8. Hashimoto thyroiditis and PTC. A grayscale ultrasound longitudinal view (*A*) of the right thyroid lobe shows a focal confluent 1.5 cm hypoechoic nodule standing out from the background of thyroiditis (*arrowheads*) with irregular borders, internal microcalcifications (*white arrows*), and mild peripheral vascularity (dashed *arrows*) on power Doppler imaging (*B*) consistent with biopsy-proven PTC. A grayscale ultrasound longitudinal view of the right lobe (*C*) and left lobe (*D*) in a different patient illustrate the diffuse hypoechoic PTC with microcalcifications (*arrows*) infiltrating the entire right lobe, in contrast with the benign heterogeneous hyperechoic Hashimoto thyroiditis of the left lobe.

the gland with homogeneously hypoechoic, lobulated contour and increase through transmission are features of PTL in underlying Hashimoto thyroiditis (**Fig. 9**).

Multinodular Goiter

Whenever facing a diffuse multinodular thyroid, it is comforting to know that an estimated 60% to 70% of thyroid nodules in which fine needle aspiration is performed are classified as benign.[11]

The majority of these represent either benign follicular nodules or thyroiditis. Benign follicular nodules comprise a range of nodules including nodular goiter, adenomatoid or hyperplastic nodules, colloid nodules, nodules of Grave's disease, and follicular adenomas, which are composed of varying proportions of benign follicular cells and colloid material on histology.[11] However, the incidence of thyroid cancer in multinodular goiter is the same and one must search for high suspicious features of the nodules as demonstrated by ATA

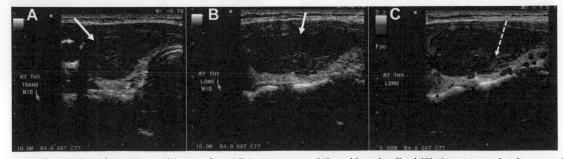

Fig. 9. Thyroid lymphoma in Hashimoto thyroiditis. Transverse (*A*) and longitudinal (*B*) view grayscale ultrasound images of the right thyroid lobe shows a 3-cm lobulated, diffusely hypoechoic nodule (*white arrows*) with increase through transmission and internal vascularity (*dashed arrow*) on power Doppler (*C*). Surgical pathology revealed B-cell lymphoma in Hashimoto thyroiditis (not shown).

and TI-RADS, as well as the detection of cystic or calcific pathologic neck lymph nodes.

Both the giraffe and the white knight patterns, associated with Hashimoto thyroiditis (as detailed in the Thyroiditis section), were previously introduced as ultrasound patterns with a 100% specificity for benignity. Additional patterns that preclude histologic confirmation include spongiform nodules and "cysts with colloid clot" associated with benign follicular nodules.[19,21] Spongiform nodules are composed of microcystic foci making up a honeycomb pattern.[25] A cyst with colloid clot refers to a cystic nodule with an avascular retracted clot with the clot having a similar honeycomb appearance to a spongiform nodule.[22] The correct identification of these patterns could obviate more than 60% of biopsies.[22]

Cross-sectional imaging, in particular CT scans, can be obtained in patients with a multinodular goiter to determine the extent of mediastinal extension not assessed by ultrasound examination (Fig. 10). This consideration is important in the preoperative evaluation of patients, as demonstrated in 1 series of 665 patients, of whom 9.5% required sternotomy for goiter resection rather than the typical cervical approach.[26] Preoperative planning with CT scan or MR imaging can more clearly define factors that would prompt the surgeon for a thoracic approach including size larger than the thoracic inlet, substernal extension or extension to the aortic arch and loss of clear plane of tissue around the goiter in the mediastinum (see Fig. 10).[26]

MALIGNANT THYROID DISEASE

Considering the vast literature on oncologic thyroid diagnosis and management, it is a daunting task to provide a comprehensive discussion of thyroid cancer. The assessment of thyroid nodules for malignant features are addressed in detail in the article of this series, titled Ultrasound of Thyroid Nodules and the Thyroid Imaging Reporting and Data System by Harshawn Malhi and Edward Grant. The following review highlights the commonly encountered thyroid malignancy with key diagnostic features and staging.

Approximately 3% to 7% of biopsied thyroid nodules are malignant with an additional 3% to 5% reported as suspicious for malignancy.[11] Primary thyroid cancer is the most common malignancy, of which 80% are PTC, with lymphoma and metastatic disease being less frequent. Thyroid follicular epithelial-derived cancers are divided into 3 major common categories: papillary (differentiated, 85%), follicular (differentiated, 12%), and anaplastic (undifferentiated, <3%). Medullary thyroid carcinoma originates from the neural crest derived parafollicular C-cells of the thyroid gland, distinguishing it as a separate category from follicular cell–derived cancers.

Local invasiveness of a thyroid nodule raises a red flag for thyroid malignancy, both clinically and radiographically, and is more commonly seen in anaplastic thyroid carcinoma, lymphoma, and sarcoma.[27] It is suggested clinically by difficulty breathing, voice changes, and dysphagia owing to involvement of the trachea and larynx, recurrent laryngeal nerve, and esophagus, respectively.[27] Cross-sectional imaging plays a critical role in delineating adjacent structural invasion, substernal extent of tumor, involvement of mediastinal structures and prevertebral space, and carotid encasement, which define resectability, surgical planning, and the potential need for sternotomy and reconstruction.[26] For example, when tumor invasion of

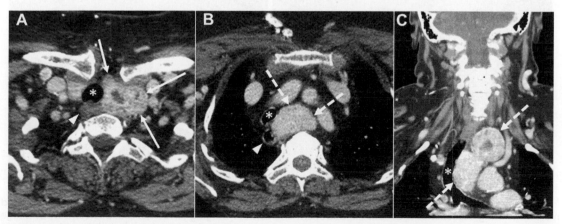

Fig. 10. Multinodular goiter. Axial (A, B) and coronal (C) postcontrast CT images of the neck show an enlarged left-sided thyroid goiter (arrow) with substernal extension into the mediastinum to the aortic arch (dashed arrows). The mediastinal component displaces the trachea (*) and esophagus (arrowhead) to the right.

the trachea extends inferiorly below the level of the sternum, the probability of the need for sternotomy increases.[28] Assessment for tracheal and/or esophageal invasion on cross-sectional imaging aids in complete presurgical evaluation to prevent incomplete resection and need for revision surgery.[28]

On imaging, local invasion is detected by extension of the tumor beyond the confines of the thyroid contour or frank invasion of neighboring structures.[27] Strap muscle involvement can be ascertained with increased certainty when the tumor extends through the muscle to the opposing surface (Fig. 11).[29] Loss of the echogenic capsule on ultrasound examination is the best predictor of the presence of extracapsular extension (T3b disease) with 75% sensitivity and 65% specificity (Fig. 12). When 3 to 4 features of capsular abutment, contour bulging, loss of echogenic capsule, and vascularity beyond the capsule are present, the specificity increases to 70% to 93% with low sensitivity of 63% to 25% (see Figs. 11 and 12). However, because T3b disease is resectable, the low sensitivity of imaging evaluation for strap muscle invasion may not be significant clinically.[30]

In the evaluation of tracheal and esophageal invasion, tumor contact of more than 180° with the trachea or esophagus, tracheal deformity, or loss of normal wall of the esophagus, or intraluminal mucosal tumor has high specificity (90%) but low sensitivity (30%–60%) (see Figs. 11 and 12).[31] The loss of the fat planes in the tracheoesophageal

groove, more than 25% of tumor abutting the capsule at the posterior thyroid and evidence of vocal cord paralysis on CT scan and/or clinical evaluation predict tumor invasion of the recurrent laryngeal nerve when at least 2 of these findings are present (see Fig. 12; Fig. 13).[31] Deformity of the common carotid artery contour and more than 180° circumferential contact with tumor increases the probability of vascular invasion, with more than 270° circumferential involvement, likely rendering the tumor unresectable.[32]

In the recent eighth edition of the American Joint Committee on Cancer staging system for differentiated thyroid cancer, notable changes were made from the seventh edition, resulting in the downstaging of many patients and included increasing the age cutoff for staging from 45 to 55 years (Table 1).[33] Microscopic invasion of tumor into adjacent soft tissues was removed as a component of T3 disease, with T3 disease now divided into T3a (>4 cm isolated to the thyroid) and T3b (any size tumor with gross ETE into strap muscles).[34] In patients 55 years of age or older, stage III disease under the eighth edition is now defined as gross invasion into subcutaneous soft tissues and posterolateral structures including the larynx, trachea, recurrent laryngeal nerve and esophagus.[33] Vascular encasement involving the carotid arteries and mediastinal arteries as well as involvement of the prevertebral fascia now define stage IVA disease.

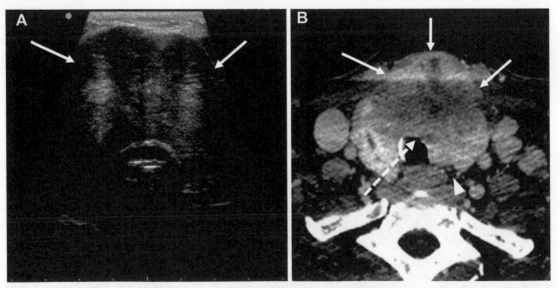

Fig. 11. Invasive PTC. Transverse grayscale ultrasound image of the thyroid gland (*A*) shows a hypoechoic solid mass infiltrating the isthmus with capsular abutment and contour bulging (*arrows*). Axial postcontrast CT image of the neck (*B*) complements findings on ultrasound and delineates anterior ETE of the mass to the strap muscles (*arrows*) and intraluminal mucosal invasion of the trachea (dashed *arrow*). Note the preservation of the tracheoesophageal groove (*arrowhead*).

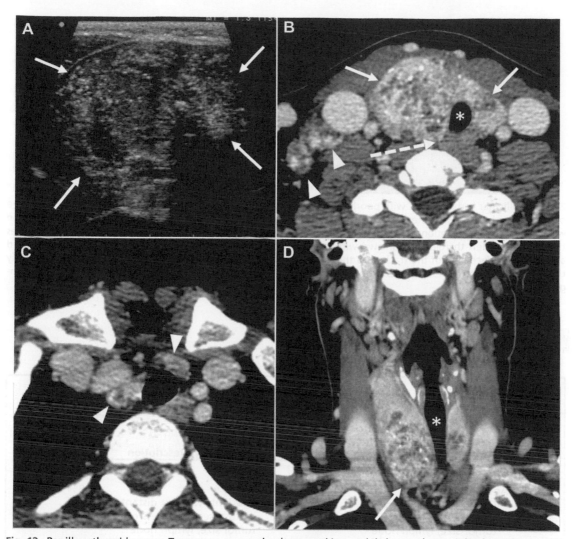

Fig. 12. Papillary thyroid cancer. Transverse gray scale ultrasound image (*A*) shows a large right thyroid lobe infiltrative hypoechoic solid mass with capsular abutment, contour bulging, and focal loss of echogenic capsule on the left (*arrows*) with numerous internal echogenic foci compatible with microcalcifications. An axial postcontrast CT scan of the neck (*B, C*) reveals a heterogeneous tumor with microcalcification centered in the right thyroid lobe with extension across the isthmus to the medial left lobe (*arrows*). There is more than 180° of tracheal abutment and displacement of the trachea to the left, suspicious for but without frank mucosal tracheal invasion (*). Posterior tumor extension and completely effaced fatty tissue in right tracheoesophageal groove (*dashed arrow*) is suspicious for tumor invasion of recurrent laryngeal nerve. The tumor abuts the right lateral aspect of the esophagus of less than 180° circumference and without esophageal invasion (*dashed arrow*). Metastatic lymphadenopathy is seen in the right lower neck (*arrowheads* in *B*) and upper mediastinum (*arrowheads* in *C*). Coronal postcontrast CT image of the neck (*D*) shows the craniocaudal dimension of the mass with inferior extension to the sternal notch (*arrow*) and displacement of the trachea to the left (*).

Papillary Thyroid Carcinoma

PTC is the most common of the differentiated thyroid cancers and has an excellent prognosis and 10-year survival rate or more than 95%.[29] In the most recent eighth edition of the AJCC staging system, patients less than 55 years of age are staged as either stage I or II, reflecting the excellent prognosis, even in the face of nodal metastases and distant metastases.[35]

Malignant thyroid lesions are more likely to be hypoechoic solid, taller than wide, and lobulated on ultrasound examination and show calcifications (American College of Radiology [ACR]-TIRAD TR5, ATA high suspicion), from 26% to 79%, versus 8% to 39% in benign lesions, with microcalcifications

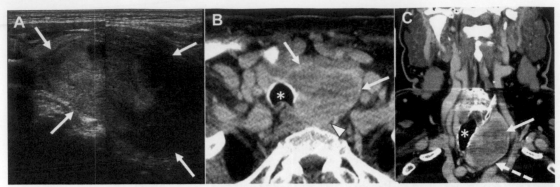

Fig. 13. Follicular variant of PTC with poorly differentiated component. Longitudinal grayscale ultrasound image of the thyroid (*A*) shows a heterogeneously hypoechoic solid nodule involving most of the left thyroid lobe without internal calcifications (*arrows*). Axial (*B*) and coronal (*C*) postcontrast CT imaging of the neck delineates the mass in the left thyroid lobe (*arrows*) with inferior extension to the upper mediastinum (*dashed arrow*) and associated displacement of the trachea to the right (*). Posterior tumor extension and completely effaced fatty tissue in the left tracheoesophageal groove (*arrowhead*) is suspicious for tumor invasion of the recurrent laryngeal nerve.

Table 1
Comparing the AJCC seventh and eighth editions for differentiated and anaplastic thyroid cancer

Stage	Seventh Edition Description	Seventh Edition 10-y DSS	Eighth Edition Description	Eighth Edition Expected 10-y DSS
Younger patients				
I	Age <45 y All patients without distant metastases regardless of tumor size, lymph node status, or ETE	97%–100%	Age <55 y All patients without distant metastases regardless of tumor size, lymph node status, or ETE	98%–100%
II	Age <45 y Distant metastases	95%–99%	Age <55 y Distant metastases	85%–95%
Older patients				
I	Age ≥45 y ≤2 cm tumor Confined to thyroid	97%–100%	Age ≥55 y ≤4 cm tumor Confined to thyroid	98%–100%
II	Age ≥45 y 2–4 cm tumor Confined to thyroid	97%–100%	Age ≥55 y Tumor >4 cm Or tumor of any size with central or lateral neck lymph nodes or gross ETE into strap muscles	85%–95%
III	Age ≥45 y >4 cm tumor Or minimal ETE or central neck lymph node metastasis	88%–95%	Age ≥55 y Tumor of any size with gross ETE into subcutaneous tissue, larynx, trachea, esophagus, recurrent laryngeal nerve	60%–70%

Adapted from Perrier ND, Brierley JD, Tuttle RM. Differentiated and anaplastic thyroid carcinoma: Major changes in the American Joint Committee on Cancer eighth edition cancer staging manual. CA Cancer J Clin. 2018;68(1):55-63. https://doi.org/10.3322/caac.21439.

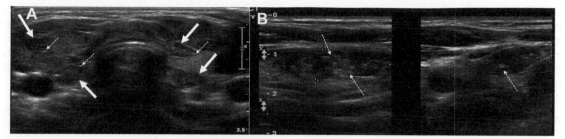

Fig. 14. A 21-year-old woman with an enlarged thyroid on physical examination. A midline transverse grayscale ultrasound image (*A*) of the thyroid shows enlargement of the gland with multifocal hypoechoic nodules in the bilateral lobes (*white arrows*) with scattered microcalcifications (dashed *arrows*). Dedicated transverse and longitudinal imaging of the right thyroid lobe (*B*) delineates one such nodule with calipers with hypoechoic echotexture and internal microcalcifications (*dashed arrows*). A biopsy revealed diffuse sclerosing variant of PTC.

more likely found in PTC (see **Figs. 11** and **12**).[4,5,32] Nodal metastases are a common occurrence in PTC and can be seen in 40% of adults diagnosed with this malignancy.[29] Metastatic lymph nodes may be cystic, necrotic, calcified or have internal hemorrhage and are well depicted on ultrasound examination.[29] Cross-sectional imaging allows for the careful evaluation of upstaging features including invasion of the trachea, esophagus, strap muscles and tumor extent for surgical planning (see **Figs. 11–13**).

The aggressive variants of PTC typically present with aggressive findings at the time of diagnosis such as ETE and metastasis as well as poorer prognosis compared with the classical PTC. In adults, they include the tall cell variant, columnar cell variant, diffuse sclerosing variant, and follicular variant.[4,5] The follicular variant typically exhibits features more commonly seen in follicular thyroid carcinoma (FTC), more likely to be isoechoic to hyperechoic, noncalcified, round nodules with regular smooth margins (see **Fig. 13**).[4,5] The tall cell variant is associated with more aggressive features, such as ETE and nodal metastases, compared with classical and follicular type PTC, and even in cases with just 10% tall cell

composition, this portends a worse prognosis including higher recurrence rates and increased mortality.[36] This variant tends to present at older age and with larger tumors compared with classical PTC.[37]

Diffuse Sclerosing Variant of Papillary Carcinoma

The diffuse sclerosing variant of papillary carcinoma is a rare, aggressive subtype that is generally diagnosed in a younger age group, particularly in female patients.[38,39] The prevalence is estimated at approximately 0.7% to 6.6% among patients with PTC.[39] This variant has a greater propensity for presenting with bilateral lesions, extracapsular extension and nodal metastases.[39] On ultrasound examination, the diffuse sclerosing variant of papillary carcinoma is characterized by diffuse enlargement of the thyroid parenchyma with heterogeneous echogenicity and numerous internal hyperechoic foci.[38] A large proportion, estimated at up to 83%, of cases show diffuse microcalcifications.[38] Additionally, 1 or multiple suspicious masses can be identified in the thyroid gland. These findings closely correlate

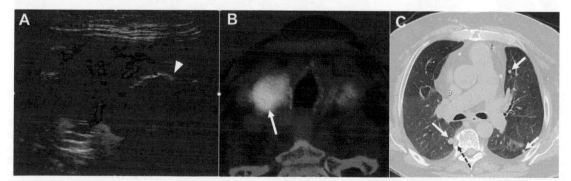

Fig. 15. FTC. Longitudinal grayscale and power Doppler ultrasound images of the thyroid (*A*) and fused axial PET-CT scan (*B*) show a lobulated hypoechoic solid hypervascular nodule in the right thyroid lobe with macrocalcification (*arrowhead* on *A*) and FDG avidity (*arrow* on *B*). Lung window axial CT imaging of the chest (*C*) shows multiple pulmonary metastasis (*white arrows*) and vertebral lytic metastasis (*dashed arrow*).

with histopathologic findings of psammoma bodies, widespread fibrosis, and lymphocytic infiltration.[38] In summary, this entity should be considered in younger adult patients with enlarged thyroids, scattered microcalcifications and suspicious masses (**Fig. 14**).[38]

Follicular Thyroid Carcinoma

FTC is the second most common type of differentiated thyroid cancer after PTC and displays a

more aggressive behavior.[40] Hematogenous metastatic spread to lung and bones may be seen in up to one-third of patients at presentation, and on pathology vascular invasion may be seen in close to one-half of patients.[41] Spread to cervical lymph nodes is uncommon compared with PTC.[29]

On ultrasound examination, FTC not only exhibits highly suspicious ultrasound features such as hypoechoic solid, lobulated/irregular margin (ACR-TIRAD TR5, ATA high suspicion), but also typically is more likely to be an isoechoic to

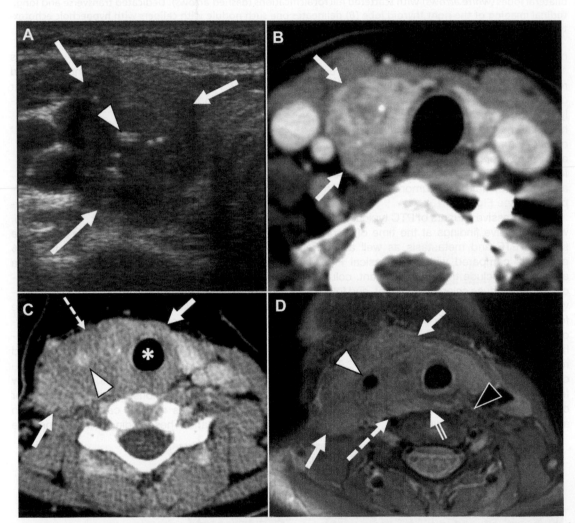

Fig. 16. Spectrum of imaging findings in medullary thyroid cancer. Patient 1 transverse grayscale ultrasound of the right thyroid lobe (*A*) shows high suspicion features of the nodule (*arrows*) include markedly hypoechoic, solid, irregular margin, taller than wide and internal calcifications (*arrowheads*). Axial postcontrast CT image of the neck of the same patient (*B*) demonstrates a heterogeneous mass with internal calcifications and without ETE (*arrows*). Patient 2 axial postcontrast CT scan of the neck (*C*) and T2 fat-saturated axial MR image (*D*) show an invasive mass in the right thyroid lobe (*arrows*) with obliteration of the internal jugular vein, and circumferential encasement/invasion of the right common carotid artery (*white arrowheads*). CT image (*C*) illustrates circumferential involvement of the trachea by hypodense tumor (***) and invasion of the strap muscles anteriorly (*dashed arrow*). MR imaging (*D*) nicely delineates how the mass posteriorly abuts the right vertebral artery (*dashed arrow*) and ventral vertebral body (*double arrow*) with invasion of the prevertebral musculature on the right and preservation on the left (*black arrowhead*).

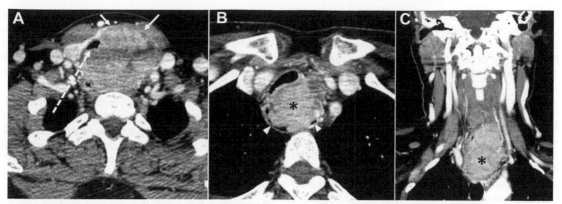

Fig. 17. Hurthle cell carcinoma. Axial (*A, B*) and coronal (*C*) postcontrast CT images of the neck show a large invasive mass centered in the left thyroid lobe with invasion of the strap muscles (*arrows*) as well as mucosal luminal invasion of the trachea (dashed *arrow*). The mass demonstrates caudal extension to the upper mediastinum (*) with gross intraluminal esophageal invasion (*arrowheads*).

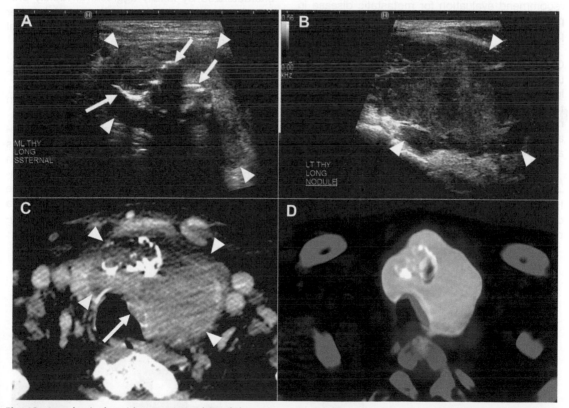

Fig. 18. Anaplastic thyroid cancer in multinodular goiter. Longitudinal grayscale ultrasound image of the isthmus (*A*) and power Doppler ultrasound image of the left lobe (*B*) show a hypoechoic mass (*arrowheads*) with calcification (*arrows*). Axial postcontrast CT image (*C*) and fusion FDG-PET/CT image (*D*) show the heterogeneous partially calcified FDG avid thyroid mass replacing the entire left thyroid lobe and isthmus (*arrowheads*) and invading the trachea (*arrow*).

hyperechoic, noncalcified, round nodule with regular smooth margins (**Fig. 15**).[4,5] Microcalcifications are less common in FTC compared with PTC, but the presence of egg shell and macrocalcifications may help to suggest FTC.[42]

Medullary Thyroid Carcinoma

Medullary thyroid cancer is rare, making up 1% to 2% of all thyroid cancers, but accounts for 13.4% of thyroid-related cancer deaths.[43] The majority of cases are sporadic, but approximately 25% cases are associated with *RET* mutations and make up part of the medullary endocrine 2A or 2B neoplasia syndromes.[44]

On ultrasound examination, most medullary thyroid cancers also exhibit the features of high and intermediate ACR TIRAD and ATA suspicion (**Fig. 16**).[45,46] The presence of microcalcification and the irregular shape of the nodule are significantly associated with metastatic lymph nodes. Medullary thyroid cancer displays aggressive behavior and, at presentation, 35% of patients have ETE or nodal disease and 13% show distant metastatic disease.[47] Current ATA guidelines recommend evaluation for metastatic disease in patients with calcitonin levels of more than 500 pg/mL.[48]

Multimodality imaging (ultrasound examination, CT scan, MR imaging, and PET/CT scan) is often used to evaluate the full extent of disease from local structural invasion, regional nodal metastasis, to distant lung and bone metastasis. Furthermore, information provided by imaging evaluation aids in determining extent of resectable disease and need for systemic treatment (see **Fig. 16**).[32]

Hurthle Cell Carcinoma

Hurthle cell carcinoma is a differentiated tumor demonstrating a more aggressive pattern of behavior compared with PTC. Previously, Hurthle cell cancer was considered a variant of follicular thyroid cancer; however, recently Hurthle cell cancer has been recognized as a distinct tumor type.[49] Like FTC, Hurthle cell thyroid cancer has a predilection for hematogenous spread to distant sites such as bone and lungs.[44]

As in other aggressive thyroid cancers, the evaluation of invasive features is important for surgical planning. ETE, including esophageal invasion with luminal disease, requires complete resection of the segment of esophageal tract involvement followed by reconstruction (**Fig. 17**).[50] When tumor invasion is confined only to the muscularis of the esophagus however, the invaded section can be resected with preservation of the underlying submucosa.[50]

Anaplastic Thyroid Carcinoma

Anaplastic (undifferentiated) carcinoma comprises 2% of primary thyroid carcinomas, most commonly occurs in people over the age of 60 years, and is characterized by locally aggressive, rapidly progressive and invasive tumors that can take over the whole lobe with a 5-month median survival rate and a 1-year survival rate of 20% (**Fig. 18**).[11] Therefore, a rapidly enlarging thyroid lobe or gland with airway compromise in adults should raise suspicion for anaplastic carcinoma.

Helpful differentiating features between anaplastic thyroid carcinoma and lymphoma on imaging include the presence of calcifications and necrosis in anaplastic thyroid carcinoma as well as heterogeneous attenuation on CT scans.[51] In contrast, lymphoma shows homogeneous attenuation and lack of calcifications and necrosis.[51] A core biopsy in suspected anaplastic thyroid carcinoma versus lymphoma can aid in initiating prompt diagnosis and treatment.

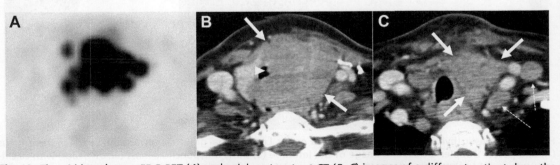

Fig. 19. Thyroid lymphoma. FDG-PET (*A*) and axial postcontrast CT (*B, C*) images of a different patient show the FDG avid, noncalcified homogenous soft tissue mass (*white arrows*) replacing the entire left thyroid lobe, invading the trachea (*arrowhead*) and associating with solid left lateral neck adenopathy (*dashed arrows*).

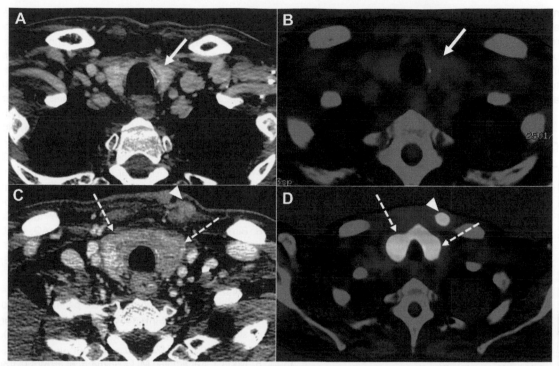

Fig. 20. Thyroid metastasis from squamous cell carcinoma of left base of tongue. Axial postcontrast CT scan of the neck (*A*) and concurrent axial fused FDG-PET/CT scan at the same level (*B*) shows a normal-sized thyroid gland with background FDG uptake (*white arrows*). Axial postcontrast CT scan of the neck (*C*) and concurrent axial fused FDG-PET/CT scan at the same level (*D*) performed 6 months later reveals interval enlargement and decreased, heterogeneous attenuation of the thyroid gland with markedly increased diffuse tracer uptake (*dashed arrows*) consistent with biopsy-proven metastatic infiltration of the thyroid gland from squamous cell carcinoma. A hypermetabolic subcutaneous nodule in the left upper chest corresponds to an additional metastatic deposit (*arrowhead*).

Thyroid Lymphoma

Thyroid lymphoma makes up 1% to 5% of thyroid malignancies and is characterized by an abnormal proliferation of lymphocytes.[11] The most common type of lymphoma to affect the thyroid is extranodal marginal zone B-cell lymphoma, followed by diffuse large B-cell lymphoma. Lymphoma of the thyroid gland generally presents as a single hypoechoic mass on ultrasound (see **Fig. 9**).[11] On CT scans, lymphoma of the solid organs often manifests as a solid enhancing mass or diffuse involvement and enlargement and can exhibit local invasiveness. The lymphomatous lymph nodes are generally enlarged and of homogeneous density (see **Fig. 16**). Non-Hodgkin lymphoma of the thyroid is a rare occurrence and generally occurs in elderly women with a prior history of Hashimoto thyroiditis or multinodular goiter. Therefore, in Hashimoto thyroiditis a confluent hypoechoic mass that is, larger than the background 0.1 to 0.6 cm micronodules, should raise suspicion for lymphoma (**Fig. 19**).[20]

To distinguish between anaplastic thyroid carcinoma or aggressive PTC and thyroid lymphoma, the radiologist must be able to identify classic lymphoma imaging features and recognize the absence of a heterogeneous multinodular thyroid gland, lack of calcifications and absence of cystic lymphadenopathy.[52]

Thyroid Metastasis

Metastasis may be due to direct invasion or distant dissemination to the thyroid and are considered rare. The most common primary tumors to metastasize to the thyroid include lung, breast and renal cell primaries (**Fig. 20**).[27] Ultrasound-guided fine-needle aspiration can be performed for histologic confirmation.[53]

SUMMARY

Imaging evaluation of the thyroid gland spans a plethora of modalities, including ultrasound examination, cross-sectional studies, and nuclear medicine techniques. The overlapping of clinical and imaging findings of benign and malignant thyroid disease can make interpretation a complex undertaking. We provide a practical approach to imaging of thyroid disease and highlight the keys to differentiate and diagnose common benign and malignant disease affecting the thyroid gland.

CLINICS CARE POINTS

- Ultrasound examination serves as the most sensitive imaging modality for evaluation of the thyroid parenchyma and for guidance of image-guided biopsies.

- Cross-sectional imaging, including CT scans and MR imaging, serves as an adjunct to assessment of thyroid pathology by providing information on disease extension and characterization of nodal stations not readily evaluated by ultrasound examination.

- The categorization of thyroid disease into diffuse and focal processes aids in narrowing the differential diagnoses.

- Entities that result in diffuse thyroid parenchymal abnormality include a broad spectrum of thyroiditis, with multinodular goiter and malignant infiltration considered within the differential considerations.

- Focal disorders of the thyroid gland include benign and malignant pathology with imaging characteristics that can guide the radiologist to favor certain entities.

- Diffuse sclerosing variant of papillary carcinoma constitutes a rare subtype that is seen in young women portends an unfavorable prognosis and is characterized by diffuse infiltration of the gland with microcalcifications and heterogeneous echogenicity.

- An underlying diagnosis of Hashimoto thyroiditis represents a risk factor for PTL and a questionable risk factor for the development of PTC.

REFERENCES

1. Chung R, Kim D. Imaging of thyroid nodules. Appl Radiol 2019;48(1):16-26.

2. Themes UFO. Cross-Sectional Imaging of the Thyroid Gland. Radiology Key. 2017. Available at: https://radiologykey.com/cross-sectional-imaging-of-the-thyroid-gland/. Accessed September 15, 2020.

3. Allen E, Fingeret A. Anatomy, Head and Neck, Thyroid. In: StatPearls [Internet]. Treasure Island (FL): StatPearls Publishing; 2021. Available at: http://www.ncbi.nlm.nih.gov/books/NBK470452/. Accessed September 15, 2020.

4. Haugen BR, Alexander EK, Bible KC, et al. 2015 American Thyroid Association Management Guidelines for Adult Patients with Thyroid Nodules and Differentiated Thyroid Cancer: the American Thyroid Association Guidelines Task Force on Thyroid Nodules and Differentiated Thyroid Cancer. Thyroid 2015;26(1):1–133.

5. Amin MB, Edge S, Greene F, et al, editors. AJCC cancer staging manual. 8th edition. Cham (Switzerland): Springer International Publishing; 2017. Available at: https://www.springer.com/gp/book/9783319406176. Accessed October 15, 2020.

6. Bin Saeedan M, Aljohani IM, Khushaim AO, et al. Thyroid computed tomography imaging: pictorial review of variable pathologies. Insights Imaging 2016; 7(4):601–17.

7. Kang T, Kim DW, Lee YJ, et al. Magnetic resonance imaging features of normal thyroid parenchyma and incidental diffuse thyroid disease: a single-center study. Front Endocrinol 2018;9. https://doi.org/10.3389/fendo.2018.00746.

8. Noda Y, Kanematsu M, Goshima S, et al. MRI of the thyroid for differential diagnosis of benign thyroid nodules and papillary carcinomas. Am J Roentgenol 2015;204(3):W332–5.

9. Sakat MS, Sade R, Kilic K, et al. The Use of Dynamic Contrast-Enhanced Perfusion MRI in Differentiating Benign and Malignant Thyroid Nodules. Indian J Otolaryngol Head Neck Surg 2019;71(Suppl 1): 706–11.

10. Wang H, Wei R, Liu W, et al. Diagnostic efficacy of multiple MRI parameters in differentiating benign vs. malignant thyroid nodules. BMC Med Imaging 2018;18(1):50.

11. Nachiappan AC, Metwalli ZA, Hailey BS, et al. The thyroid: review of imaging features and biopsy techniques with radiologic-pathologic correlation. RadioGraphics 2014;34(2):276–93.

12. Sundram F. Clinical use of PET/CT in thyroid cancer diagnosis and management. Biomed Imaging Interv J 2006;2(4).

13. Ahuja AT, Ying M. Sonographic evaluation of cervical lymph nodes. Am J Roentgenol 2005;184(5):1691–9.

14. Sohn Y-M, Kwak JY, Kim E-K, et al. Diagnostic approach for evaluation of lymph node metastasis from thyroid cancer using ultrasound and fine-needle aspiration biopsy. Am J Roentgenol 2010; 194(1):38–43.

15. Sweeney LB, Stewart C, Gaitonde DY. Thyroiditis: an integrated approach. Am Fam Physician 2014;90(6): 389–96.

16. Yuen HY, Wong KT, Ahuja AT. Sonography of diffuse thyroid disease. Australas J Ultrasound Med 2016; 19(1):13–29.

17. Cappelli C, Pirola I, Martino ED, et al. The role of imaging in Graves' disease: a cost-effectiveness analysis. Eur J Radiol 2008. https://doi.org/10.1016/j.ejrad.2007.03.015.

18. Intenzo CM, dePapp AE, Jabbour S, et al. Scintigraphic Manifestations of Thyrotoxicosis. RadioGraphics 2003;23(4):857–69.

19. Charkes ND, Maurer AH, Siegel JA, et al. MR imaging in thyroid disorders: correlation of signal intensity with Graves disease activity. Radiology 1987;164:491–4.

20. Yeh HC, Futterweit W, Gilbert P. Micronodulation: ultrasonographic sign of Hashimoto thyroiditis. J Ultrasound Med 1996;15(12):813–9.

21. Virmani V, Hammond I. Sonographic patterns of benign thyroid nodules: verification at our institution. Am J Roentgenol 2011;196(4):891–5.

22. Bonavita JA, Mayo J, Babb J, et al. Pattern recognition of benign nodules at ultrasound of the thyroid: which nodules can be left alone? Am J Roentgenol 2009;193(1):207–13.

23. Graceffa G, Patrone R, Vieni S, et al. Association between Hashimoto's thyroiditis and papillary thyroid carcinoma: a retrospective analysis of 305 patients. BMC Endocr Disord 2019;19(Suppl 1). https://doi.org/10.1186/s12902-019-0351-x.

24. Mehta K, Liu C, Raad RA, et al. Thyroid lymphoma: a case report and literature review. World J Otorhinolaryngol 2015;5(3):82–9.

25. Moon W-J, Jung SL, Lee JH, et al. Benign and malignant thyroid nodules: US differentiation—multicenter retrospective study. Radiology 2008;247(3):762–70.

26. Coskun A, Yildirim M, Erkan N. Substernal goiter: when is a sternotomy required? Int Surg 2014;99(4):419–25.

27. Hoang JK, Lee WK, Lee M, et al. US features of thyroid malignancy: pearls and pitfalls. RadioGraphics 2007;27(3):847–60.

28. Tran J, Zafereo M. Segmental tracheal resection (nine rings) and reconstruction for carcinoma showing thymus-like differentiation (CASTLE) of the thyroid. Head Neck 2019;41(9):3478–81.

29. Hoang JK, Sosa JA, Nguyen XV, et al. Imaging thyroid disease: updates, imaging approach, and management pearls. Radiol Clin North Am 2015;53(1):145–61.

30. Kamaya A, Tahvildari AM, Patel BN, et al. Sonographic detection of extracapsular extension in papillary thyroid cancer. J Ultrasound Med 2015;34(12):2225–30.

31. Seo YL, Yoon DY, Lim KJ, et al. Locally advanced thyroid cancer: can CT help in prediction of extrathyroidal invasion to adjacent structures? AJR Am J Roentgenol 2010;195(3):W240–4.

32. Traylor KS. Computed Tomography and MR Imaging of Thyroid Disease. Radiol Clin North Am 2020;58(6):1059–70.

33. Perrier ND, Brierley JD, Tuttle RM. Differentiated and anaplastic thyroid carcinoma: major changes in the American Joint Committee on Cancer eighth edition cancer staging manual. CA Cancer J Clin 2018;68(1):55–63.

34. Tam S, Boonsripitayanon M, Amit M, et al. Survival in differentiated thyroid cancer: comparing the AJCC Cancer Staging Seventh and Eighth Editions. Thyroid 2018;28(10):1301–10.

35. Shaha AR, Migliacci JC, Nixon IJ, et al. Stage migration with the new American Joint Committee on Cancer (AJCC) staging system (8th edition) for differentiated thyroid cancer. Surgery 2019;165(1):6–11.

36. Vuong HG, Long NP, Anh NH, et al. Papillary thyroid carcinoma with tall cell features is as aggressive as tall cell variant: a meta-analysis. Endocr Connect 2018;7(12):R286–93.

37. Cartwright S, Fingeret A. Contemporary evaluation and management of tall cell variant of papillary thyroid carcinoma. Curr Opin Endocrinol Diabetes Obes 2020;27(5):351–7.

38. Kwak JY, Kim E-K, Hong SW, et al. Diffuse sclerosing variant of papillary carcinoma of the thyroid: ultrasound features with histopathological correlation. Clin Radiol 2007;62(4):382–6.

39. Chereau N, Giudicelli X, Pattou F, et al. Diffuse sclerosing variant of papillary thyroid carcinoma is associated with aggressive histopathological features and a poor outcome: results of a large multicentric study. J Clin Endocrinol Metab 2016;101(12):4603–10.

40. Gillanders SL, O'Neill JP. Prognostic markers in well differentiated papillary and follicular thyroid cancer (WDTC). Eur J Surg Oncol 2018;44(3):286–96.

41. Grani G, Lamartina L, Durante C, et al. Follicular thyroid cancer and Hürthle cell carcinoma: challenges in diagnosis, treatment, and clinical management. Lancet Diabetes Endocrinol 2018;6(6):500–14.

42. Kuo T-C, Wu M-H, Chen K-Y, et al. Ultrasonographic features for differentiating follicular thyroid carcinoma and follicular adenoma. Asian J Surg 2020;43(1):339–46.

43. Chen L, Qian K, Guo K, et al. A Novel N Staging System for Predicting Survival in Patients with Medullary Thyroid Cancer. Ann Surg Oncol 2019;26(13):4430–8.

44. Cabanillas ME, McFadden DG, Durante C. Thyroid cancer. Lancet 2016;388(10061):2783–95.

45. Yun G, Kim YK, Choi SI, et al. Medullary thyroid carcinoma: application of Thyroid Imaging Reporting and Data System (TI-RADS) Classification. Endocrine 2018;61(2):285–92.

46. Hahn SY, Shin JH, Oh YL, et al. Ultrasonographic characteristics of medullary thyroid carcinoma according to nodule size: application of the Korean Thyroid Imaging Reporting and Data System and American Thyroid

Association guidelines. Acta Radiol 2020. https://doi.org/10.1177/0284185120929699. 284185120929699.

47. Kushchayev SV, Kushchayeva YS, Tella SH, et al. Medullary thyroid carcinoma: an update on imaging. J Thyroid Res 2019;2019:1893047.

48. Wells SA, Asa SL, Dralle H, et al. Revised American Thyroid Association guidelines for the management of medullary thyroid carcinoma. Thyroid 2015; 25(6):567–610.

49. Kakudo K, Bychkov A, Bai Y, et al. The new 4th edition World Health Organization classification for thyroid tumors, Asian perspectives. Pathol Int 2018;68. https://doi.org/10.1111/pin.12737.

50. Metere A, Aceti V, Giacomelli L. The surgical management of locally advanced well-differentiated thyroid carcinoma: changes over the years according to the AJCC 8th edition Cancer Staging Manual. Thyroid Res 2019;12:10.

51. Ahmed S, Ghazarian MP, Cabanillas ME, et al. Imaging of anaplastic thyroid carcinoma. AJNR Am J Neuroradiol 2018;39(3):547–51.

52. Johnson SA, Kumar A, Matasar MJ, et al. Imaging for staging and response assessment in lymphoma. Radiology 2015;276(2):323–38.

53. Debnam JM, Kwon M, Fornage BD, et al. Sonographic evaluation of intrathyroid metastases. J Ultrasound Med 2017;36(1):69–76.

Ultrasound of Thyroid Nodules and the Thyroid Imaging Reporting and Data System

Harshawn S. Malhi, MD[a],*, Edward G. Grant, MD[b]

KEYWORDS

- Thyroid • Thyroid nodules • TIRADS • Radiology • Thyroid imaging • Thyroid cancer • Ultrasound

KEY POINTS

- Ultrasound has emerged as the optimal noninvasive imaging modality in helping to determine which thyroid nodules demonstrate suspicious features of malignancy, and thus warrant further evaluation with fine needle aspiration biopsy.
- In 2017, the American College of Radiology Thyroid Imaging Reporting and Data System committee published a white paper with a standardized (lexicon) approach to classifying nodules on ultrasound, termed Thyroid Imaging Reporting and Data System.
- Because a majority of thyroid nodules are benign, applying the Thyroid Imaging Reporting and Data System results in a meaningful decrease in the number of thyroid nodules biopsied and significantly improves the specificity of cancer detection, without sacrificing sensitivity.

INTRODUCTION

Thyroid nodules are common in the general adult population. It is estimated that approximately 60% of adults have a thyroid nodule, the majority of which are asymptomatic, nonpalpable and incidentally found on imaging such as ultrasound (US) examination, computed tomography scans, and MR imaging. Most thyroid nodules are benign; a malignancy is present in only 5% to 7% of nodules. Thus, to avoid overtreatment, it is imperative to determine which nodules are benign versus malignant. Currently, fine needle aspiration biopsy (FNAB) is considered the gold standard in determining if a nodule is malignant or will require eventual surgical resection to determine definitive pathologic diagnosis. Given the sheer number of nodules, performing FNAB on every nodule is impractical. Thyroid US imaging has emerged at the imaging modality of choice in helping to determine which nodules possess certain characteristics seen with malignancy and ultimately which nodules should or should not be biopsied. In addition to briefly reviewing thyroid nodule epidemiology and pathology, this article focuses on those specific features seen on thyroid US examination, which help to distinguish between malignancy and benignity within nodules and how these characteristics have shaped the creation of the Thyroid Imaging Reporting and Data System (TIRADS), a standardized risk stratification system for thyroid nodules purposed by the American College of Radiology (ACR).

EPIDEMIOLOGY

The worldwide incidence of thyroid cancer was estimated to represent 5.1% of all cancers in

[a] Department of Radiology, Keck School of Medicine, University of Southern California, 1500 San Pablo Street, Second Floor Imaging, Los Angeles, CA 90033, USA; [b] USC, Keck USC Hospital, 1500 San Pablo Street, Los Angeles, CA 90033, USA
* Corresponding author.
E-mail address: Harshawn.malhi@med.usc.edu

Neuroimag Clin N Am 31 (2021) 285–300
https://doi.org/10.1016/j.nic.2021.04.001
1052-5149/21/© 2021 Elsevier Inc. All rights reserved.

2018.[1] In the United States, the incidence has increased to become 3.3% of all cancers diagnosed in 2012, previously 1.0% in 1975.[2,3] Patients less than 15 years of age and more than 45 years of age have a higher probability of a thyroid nodule being malignant as well as nodules found in men compared with women. Palpable thyroid nodules occur in only 3% to 7% of adults, with 6.4% of palpable nodules present in females versus only 1.5% in males.[4] Known risk factors for developing thyroid cancer include childhood radiation exposure in the form of radioactive fallout or radiotherapy, including low-dose treatment for benign conditions; hereditary syndromes associated with thyroid cancer (eg, multiple endocrine neoplasia syndrome type 2A, Carney complex, Werner syndrome); and a family history of thyroid cancer.[5,6] In general, there has been an increasing incidence of thyroid cancer diagnoses but an overall decreased global mortality, most likely owing to earlier detection of small indolent papillary thyroid carcinoma (PTC).[2,3] The increased incidence has in part been due to greater diagnostic detection with US examination and subsequent FNAB of smaller lesions that in years past would not have been biopsied.[7] This uptrending incidence is also attributed to incidental thyroid nodule detection on increasing usage of cross-sectioning imaging modalities, such as computed tomography scans and MR imaging, with those discovered nodules then being referred for further evaluation with US imaging.[8] Recent studies have also associated in increasing incidence of thyroid cancer with a combination of environmental factors and metabolic disturbances, such as the increasing prevalence of diabetes and the metabolic syndrome in the general population.[9]

Overdiagnosis of thyroid cancer is defined as "diagnosis of thyroid tumors that would not, if left alone, result in symptoms or death."[10] In the United States, between 2003 and 2007, overdiagnosis accounted for 45% of cases in men and 70% to 80% of cases for women.[3,9] Overdiagnosis may be detrimental secondary to the physical, psychological, and financial burdens associated with the extra diagnostic testing and surgery.[11,12] Fortunately, the incidence of thyroid cancer has plateaued over the past few years, suggesting the upward trend is stabilizing.[3,12–14]

OVERVIEW OF THYROID NODULES

The thyroid gland is composed of follicular cells surrounded by colloid. When there is a proliferation of either follicular cells or colloid, a nodule will develop. From a radiologic standpoint, a thyroid nodule is a discrete lesion within the gland that is distinct from the surrounding thyroid parenchyma.[15] In nodules evaluated by FNAB, approximately 60% to 70% are benign and most commonly represent benign follicular nodules or thyroiditis.[16] The Bethesda system was devised in 2007 as a 6-tiered classification system for cytology reporting of thyroid FNAB results.[17] The 6 categories, along with the associated risk of malignancy, include (I) nondiagnostic (1%–4%), (II) benign (0%–3%), (III) atypia of undetermined significance or follicular lesion of undetermined significance (5%–15%), (IV) follicular neoplasm (15%–30%), (V) suspicious for malignancy (65%–75%), and (VI) malignant (97%–99%). Benign is the most common Bethesda calcification assigned, representing 60% to 70% of all FNAB cytology reports.[16,17]

Benign thyroid nodules

Follicular nodules are composed predominately of benign appearing follicular cells and colloid in various proportions and are usually treated nonsurgically with clinical follow-up, unless they are symptomatic from mass effect owing to size. Subtypes include adenomatoid or hyperplastic nodules, colloid nodules, nodular goiter, and macrofollicular subtype follicular adenoma. It is important to note that these various benign subtypes cannot be distinguished at FNAB alone.[18–20] Thyroiditis represents inflammation of the thyroid gland. Subtypes include Riedel (fibrous) thyroiditis, de Quervain (granulomatous or subacute) thyroiditis, acute infectious thyroiditis, and chronic lymphocytic thyroiditis (including Hashimoto's thyroiditis and autoimmune or Graves' disease). In general, thyroiditis is not biopsied, but some types can present with a nodular appearance akin to a "giraffe pattern," for example, Hashimoto's thyroiditis[20,21] (Fig. 1).

Follicular adenoma is a proliferation of follicular cells surrounded by a complete capsule. On surgical pathology, it is benign, but it is indeterminate on FNAB cytology as the presence of capsular invasion, as seen with follicular carcinoma (FC), cannot be determined. For this reason, FNAB of either a follicular adenoma or FC may generate a cytology report of either follicular lesion of undetermined significance (Bethesda III) or follicular neoplasm (Bethesda IV) and a repeat FNAB or surgical hemithyroidectomy is indicated to establish definitive pathology. Recently, genetic or molecular testing of the biopsy material has become a common, noninvasive alternative to repeat biopsy or surgery.[18] These tests assess the biopsy material for various genetic mutations associated with cancer and typically provide an estimate of the

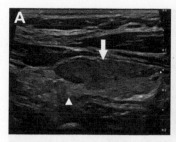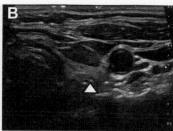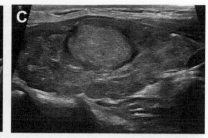

Fig. 1. (A–C), Hashimoto's thyroiditis. (A, B) Longitudinal and transverse images through the left lobe of the thyroid show an atrophied thyroid with parenchymal heterogeneity (*white arrow*) and severe surface scarring. There is often echogenic tissue surrounding such glands (*white arrowheads*). They should not be confused with a nodule. (C) A "giraffe pattern": Multiple confluent echogenic nodules are another pattern seen with Hashimoto's and are "leave alone lesions."

likelihood of malignancy in the nodule in question, ranging from low to high suspicion, thus providing guidance for the decision-making process of whether to follow the nodule or intervene surgically.[5] A nodule reported as follicular neoplasm at FNAB has a 70% to 85% chance of being a benign follicular adenoma and a 15% to 30% chance of being malignant. A variant of follicular adenoma is a Hürthle cell adenoma, in which more than 75% of cells demonstrate oncocytic or Hürthle cell changes. On cytologic analysis, Hürthle cells can be mistaken for similar appearing cells such as medullary thyroid cancer (MTC), parathyroid cells, and benign macrophages.[18,20]

Malignant thyroid nodules

Most thyroid malignancies are primary thyroid carcinomas, which include PTC, FC, MTC, and anaplastic carcinoma (AC). PTC and FC have a relatively good prognosis, MTC an intermediate prognosis, and AC a poor prognosis.[20,22] Secondary malignant lesions include metastatic disease and lymphoma. In general, malignant thyroid nodules share common imaging features on US imaging: solid, hypoechoic, lobulated or spiculated margins and internal echogenic foci (see the TIRADS section).[23] PTC represents 81% of all primary thyroid malignancies. Total thyroidectomy or lobectomy (for some lesions <3 cm) is usually performed when FNAB is diagnostic for PTC, with or without subsequent radioactive iodine ablation[20,22] (Fig. 2).

FC represents 12% of all primary thyroid malignancies and is more commonly found in older male patients. Total thyroidectomy is the treatment of choice for invasive cancer, with or without subsequent radioactive iodine ablation. Lobectomy or isthmusectomy are used for minimally invasive disease. Hürthle cell carcinoma is a variant of FC in which more than 75% of cells show oncocytic or Hürthle cell changes. The propensity for locoregional nodal metastasis with this variant may be higher than for standard FC.[20,22,24,25] US features cannot reliably distinguish between FC and follicular adenoma, but some findings to suggest carcinoma include increasing lesion volume, lack of a sonographic halo, hypoechoic appearance, and the absence of internal cystic changes[26] (Fig. 3).

MTC represents 5% of all primary thyroid malignancy and is derived from thyroid parafollicular neuroendocrine C cells that secrete calcitonin.[27] Familial conditions such as multiple endocrine neoplasia syndrome type 2A are associated with 20% of MTC cases, with the other 80% being sporadic. Because they derive from C cells, MTCs do not concentrate iodine and, as such, ^{131}I scintigraphy and radioactive iodine ablation does not play a role in the diagnosis and treatment of these carcinomas.[20] Although MTCs and PTCs share overlapping features on US imaging, MTCs tend to be larger, more cystic, and have a more homogeneous echotexture within the solid component of the lesion. Macrocalcifications are the most common echogenic foci seen in MTC[28,29] (Fig. 4).

AC accounts for 2% of all primary thyroid malignancies and portends a poor prognosis given its highly malignant nature, representing more than 50% of deaths from thyroid cancer.[18,30] Because of its usually wide local invasion, surgery is rarely an option. Like MTC, ACs do not concentrate iodine, thus precluding the use of ^{131}I scintigraphy and radioactive iodine ablation.[20] The US features of AC are nonspecific but include a large, heterogenous, solid mass with internal vascularity.[31] AC should be considered in the differential diagnosis of any rapidly enlarging thyroid mass, along with lymphoma.[32] Contrast-enhanced computed tomography scans are useful in evaluating the extension and invasion of AC into the adjacent neck structures[33–35] (Fig. 5).

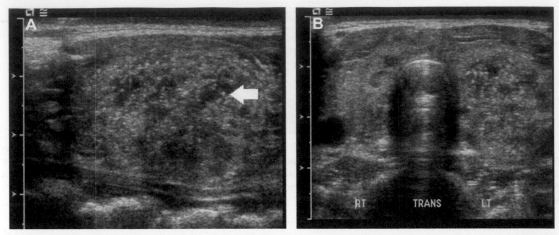

Fig. 2. (*A, B*) Papillary carcinoma. (*A, B*) Longitudinal and transverse images from a 27-year-old woman with a neck mass. The left lobe is essentially replaced by a solid mass containing innumerable punctate echogenic foci, TIRADS 5 (TR5) (*white arrow*).

Thyroid lymphoma is usually of the non-Hodgkin's type and is uncommon.[36] It may present as a primary thyroid tumor (usually in the setting of Hashimoto's thyroiditis) or as a component of generalized lymphoma.[23,37] The US features are nonspecific and similar to those seen in other primary thyroid malignancies, save for the fact that they usually do not contain echogenic foci or calcifications[38,39] (Fig. 6).

Metastases to the thyroid are rare and usually originate from renal cell carcinoma, breast, or lung primary malignancies. Metastatic disease should be suspected in a new or enlarging thyroid nodule in a patient with a known primary malignancy[20,23,40,41] (Fig. 7).

THE THYROID IMAGING, REPORTING AND DATA SYSTEM

Thyroid US examination has emerged as the first-line tool in the risk stratification of thyroid nodules.

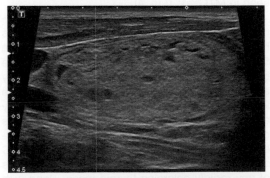

Fig. 3. FC. Large solid well-defined isoechoic mass without calcifications is identified in this 48-year-old man, TIRADS 4 (TR4). FNA results were initially follicular neoplasm (Bethesda VI) and genetic testing was suspicious. Surgery revealed FC.

US imaging is relatively cost effective, noninvasive, without ionizing radiation, and easily accessible, and the high-resolution linear probe provides for excellent visualization of the superficially located gland.[42,43] As mentioned in the Introduction, it is impractical to perform a FNAB all thyroid nodules. Thus, US examination has emerged as a reliable and noninvasive method to screen which nodules warrant biopsy based on their specific US features. Several professional societies and researchers have developed methods to aid practitioners in recommending FNAB based on certain US features of nodules, with the aim to improve patient management and cost effectiveness by avoiding unnecessary FNABs.[5,44,45] The lack of congruity within these systems as to which nodules should be biopsied, however, has limited the adaption of any single system by the US community.

The ACR TIRADS committee in 2017 published a white paper with a standardized (lexicon) approach to classifying nodules, termed TIRADS, which was modeled in a similar manner to the ACR's Breast Imaging Reporting and Data Systems, a system that has gained wide acceptance and use in breast imaging. Based on the US features of a nodule, points are assigned, with more points being assigned to more suspicious appearing nodules.[46] The summation of these points results in the nodule being placed into 1 of 5 lexicon categories: #1 benign, #2 not suspicious, #3 minimally suspicious, #4 moderately suspicious, and #5 highly suspicious for malignancy. When evaluating a nodule, the reader selects one feature from each of the first 4 categories and all the features that apply for the final category and sums up the points. The total number of points

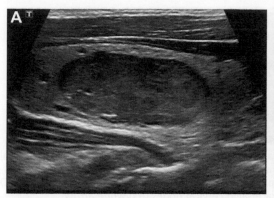

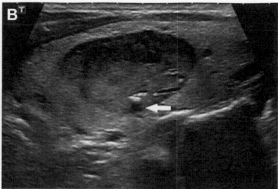

Fig. 4. (*A, B*) Medullary carcinoma. Longitudinal and transverse images from a 46-year-old woman show a solid, smoothly marginated, hypoechoic mass in the left lobe, TIRADS 4 (TR4). Note shadowing macrocalcifications posteriorly (*white arrow*). The patient had no predisposing conditions. FNA indicated medullary carcinoma, which was confirmed at surgery.

determines the nodule's TIRADS level, which ranges from TIRADS 1 (TR1—benign) to TIRADS 5 (TR5—high suspicion of malignancy). Recommendations for FNA or US follow-up are based on the nodule's TIRADS level and its maximum diameter (**Fig. 8**). Lower size limits were also defined for recommending US follow-up on TIRADS 3 (TR3), TIRADS (TR4), and TR5 nodules to limit repeat US examinations on those lesions that are likely to be benign and/or not clinically significant. In general, in keeping with the recommendations of other groups,[5] the committee strived to recommend biopsy of suspicious appearing nodules only if they are greater than 1 cm. They also

advocated biopsy of nodules only if they measure 2.5 cm or greater for TR 3 nodules and 1.5 cm for TR 4 nodules.[43,46]

Categories

Composition

The internal components of the nodule, specifically the proportion of the nodule that demonstrates the presence of fluid or soft tissue, defines the composition.[47] A nodule being classified in this area should fit into one of 4 categories in TIRADS (**Fig. 9**). Cystic or almost completely cystic thyroid nodules usually represent colloid nodules and have a very low risk of malignancy.[48]

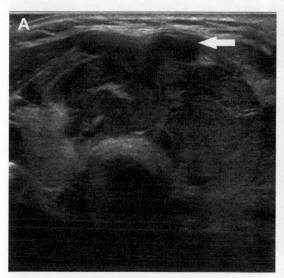

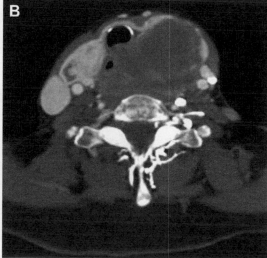

Fig. 5. (*A, B*) AC. (*A*) Transverse ultrasound image shows a large solid mass extending across the midline and apparently invading the surrounding soft tissues, TIRADS 5 (TR5) (*white arrow*). (*B*) A computed tomography scan confirms the ultrasound findings and can be particularly helpful in advanced cases such as this to define anatomy before surgery.

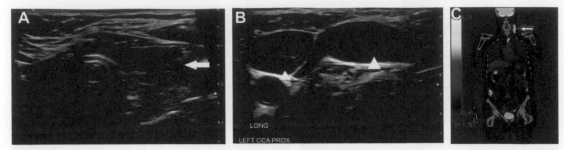

Fig. 6. (*A–C*) Thyroid lymphoma. (*A*) A solid hypoechoic mass was identified in the thyroid and biopsy was typical of lymphoma, TIRADS 4 (TR4) (*white arrowheads*). The ultrasound features are not specific. (*B*) Extensive perithyroidal adenopathy was present (*white arrowhead*). The patient had no history of Hashimoto's thyroiditis. (*C*) Whole body positron emission tomography scan shows tracer-avid cervical nodes (*red/white arrow*).

Mixed cystic and solid nodules confer a score of 1 point in the composition category (a lesser association with malignancy), whereas a solid or almost completely solid nodule should receive 2 points (a greater association with malignancy). Because these nodules present as a continuum, distinguishing solid nodules from mixed cystic and solid nodules may be difficult in everyday practice. In general, however, to receive a classification of solid or almost completely solid, less than approximately 5% of the nodule should contain cystic spaces. It should be noted that PTCs are usually solid; however, some can undergo necrosis or cystic degeneration. One study evaluating mixed cystic and solid nodules showed that the prevalence of malignancy was low regardless of whether the nodule was mostly cystic (6.1%) or mostly solid (5.7%).[49] When characterizing mixed

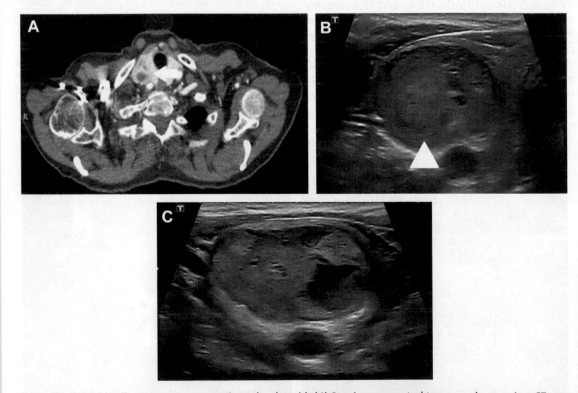

Fig. 7. (*A–C*) Renal cell carcinoma metastatic to the thyroid. (*A*) Staging computed tomography scan in a 67-year-old man with a large right renal mass consistent with renal cell carcinoma (not shown), with an incidentally noted heterogenous right thyroid nodule (*white arrow*). (*B, C*). Transverse and longitudinal ultrasound images show a smoothly marginated cystic and solid mass in the right lobe of the thyroid, TIRADS 3 (TR3) (*arrowhead*). The ultrasound features are not specific, but FNA confirmed metastatic clear cell renal carcinoma.

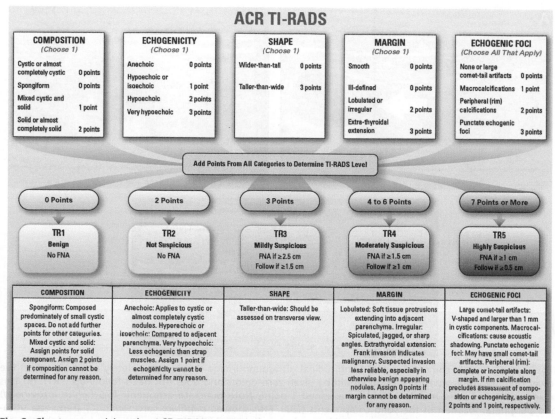

Fig. 8. Chart summarizing the ACR-TIRADS system. (*From* ACR Thyroid Imaging, Reporting and Data System (TI-RADS): White paper of the ACR TI-RADS Committee. Tessler FN, Middleton WR, Grant EG et al. JACR 2017; 14: 587-595.)

cystic and solid nodules, it is essential to evaluate the solid components. The risk for malignancy increases when the solid component has certain features, such as being eccentrically or peripherally located within the partially cystic nodule. In addition, the risk of malignancy increases if the solid aspect of the nodule has an irregular border, contains echogenic foci, and is hypoechoic. Conversely, if the solid portion of the nodule is located more centrally within the nodule, is spongiform in appearance, contains comet tail artifacts and possesses a smooth margin, it is likely to be benign. Finally, color or power Doppler interrogation of nodules has not been shown to discriminate between malignant or benign nodules reliably and, for that reason, was not included in the overall TIRADS evaluation of nodules. Discovering internal vascularity within the solid component of a nodule, however, is useful in distinguishing it from debris, hemorrhagic material, clots, and necrosis.[43,50,51]

A final note is warranted on spongiform nodules, which demonstrate the presence of very small cysts akin to a fluid filled space of a wet sponge

(**Fig. 10**). Nodules classified as spongiform are considered benign with no further follow-up required per TIRADS (TR1). At least 50% of the nodule volume should be occupied by tiny cysts before being classified as a spongiform nodule. The presence of other features such as peripheral or shadowing macrocalcifications should preclude any characterization of a spongiform nodule.[46,47]

Echogenicity

Defined as the nodule's reflectivity of the noncalcified, solid component relative to the surrounding thyroid tissue, echogenicity is divided into 4 categories[47] (**Fig. 11**). There is an association with nodule echogenicity and nodule malignancy. In general, hypoechoic nodules have a higher rate of malignancy then nodules that are isoechoic or hyperechoic.[52] Very hypoechoic nodules have very high specificity for malignancy but are not very common, whereas hypoechoic nodules are more sensitive for malignancy but less specific.[53] The solid component of a nodule's echogenicity should be compared with adjacent normal appearing thyroid parenchyma when possible. This

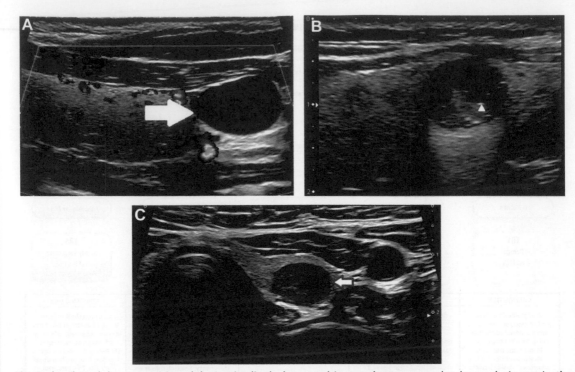

Fig. 9. (A–C) Nodule composition. (A) Longitudinal ultrasound image shows a completely anechoic cyst in the lower pole (*white arrow*). This lesion would be given zero points and does not need follow-up (TR1). (B) This mixed cystic and solid nodule would be assigned 1 point. Note punctate echogenic foci (*white arrowhead*) and peripheral location of the solid components (TR4). FNA showed papillary carcinoma. (C) Transverse ultrasound image shows a smooth bordered solid hypoechoic nodule in the lower pole of the left lobe of the thyroid (TR4) (*red/white arrow*). FNA results suggested a Hurthle cell lesion (Bethesda IV). Genetic test results were low suspicion. The lesion has been followed with ultrasound imaging and is stable.

guideline applies even if the background thyroid parenchyma is abnormal, such as that seen in chronic or acute thyroiditis. In those situations, however, a note should be made describing the altered background echogenicity. If the solid

Fig. 10. pongiform nodule: A 4.5-cm mass in the right lobe of the thyroid is essentially completely spongiform in appearance (TR1) (*white arrow*). Unlike the American Thyroid Association guidelines, the ACR TI-RADS does not recommend biopsy of spongiform lesions, regardless of size.

portion of the nodule demonstrates mixed echogenicity, then the point category assigned should be that of the predominant echogenicity.[43]

Of note, various scanning parameters can alter the relative reflectivity of nodules, something that can affect the designation of anechoic/cystic, hypoechoic and very hypoechoic nodules, as such nodules can seem to be similar. This point is important, in that cystic or almost completely cystic nodules warrant an anechoic or zero-point designation, whereas hypoechoic nodules a score of 2 points and very hypoechoic a score of 3 points. Specifically, gain, compression, transmit frequency, and preprocessing and postprocessing can alter the reflectivity of nodules. Evaluating these problematic nodules with different gain, multiple planes of section, and with real-time cine clips may be of value.[43] In addition, if the nodule is more hypoechoic than the adjacent neck strap muscles, it should be classified as very hypoechoic. The presence of posterior acoustic enhancement and a lack of internal vascular flow can help to distinguish a nodule that is a completely anechoic cyst mimicking a hypoechoic solid nodule. Because

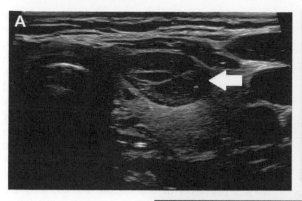
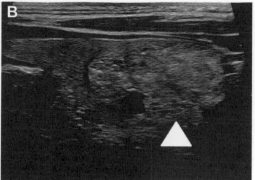
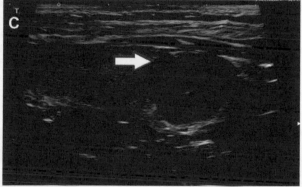

Fig. 11. (*A–C*) Nodule echogenicity. (*A*) Hypoechoic mixed cystic and solid mass in upper pole of the left thyroid. Features were that of a TR3 greater than 2.5 cm lesion (*white arrow*). FNA indicated a benign colloid nodule (Bethesda II). (*B*) Hyperechoic, solid mass in left lobe of thyroid with punctate echogenic foci (*white arrowhead*). Thee features were consistent with a TR4 lesion. FNA results were a benign follicular nodule (Bethesda II). (*C*) Very hypoechoic solid mass in the left lower pole, TR5. Note lobulated margins (*red/white arrow*). Very hypoechoic lesions are by definition less echogenic that the adjacent strap muscles. FNA revealed a papillary carcinoma (Bethesda VI).

both isoechoic and hyperechoic nodules receive 1 point in TIRADS, distinguishing between these 2 categories is not as imperative.

Finally, a nodule containing a large obscuring shadowing calcification can make determining the true internal echogenicity challenging. It is safe to assume that in such situations the nodule will be at minimum hyperechoic or isoechoic and should therefore receive at least 1 point in this category.[46,47]

Shape

A taller than wide shape of a nodule is defined as a ratio of greater than 1 in the anteroposterior diameter to the horizontal diameter when measured in the transverse plane.[47] This taller shape is a highly specific indicator of malignancy, but relatively insensitive. Given the high association with malignancy, 3 points are assigned to these nodules (**Fig. 12**). Twelve percent of nodules are found to demonstrate this appearance, and the notion of decreased compressibility is thought to be the underlying pathologic process.[54] Measurements can

be made for confirmation, but often these nodules are readily apparent on first impression. The key is to distinguish which nodules are more suspicious appearing by having possibly violated tissue planes by growing in a more front-to-back than side-to side manner. Finally, it is acceptable to classify nodules that are perfectly round as wider than tall and not taller than wide.[43,55–57]

Margin

Margin is defined as the appearance of the interface or border between the nodule and neighboring thyroid parenchyma or adjacent extrathyroidal structures.[47] Classification is divided into 4 subcategories (**Fig. 13**). Smooth borders present as even and uninterrupted and typically confer an elliptical or spherical shape and receive 0 points. Irregular margins are those that are jagged, spiculated, and with sharp angles with or without clear soft tissue protrusions into the adjacent thyroid parenchyma. These protrusions may be focal or diffuse and vary in size and conspicuity; this appearance warrants a score of 2

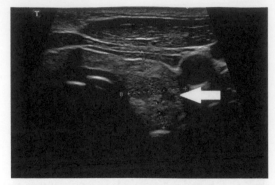

Fig. 12. Taller than wide nodule. Section taken in the transverse plane reveals a solid isoechoic nodule with punctate echogenic foci that is taller than wide both visually and by measurement (*white arrow*). Biopsy revealed a papillary carcinoma (Bethesda VI).

points. Lobulated borders have a focal soft tissue protrusion extending into the adjacent thyroid parenchyma and such nodules also receive 2 points. As with irregular margins, lobulations can be multiple or single and can vary in size and conspicuity. Of note, small lobulations are sometimes referred to as "microlobulated".

If a nodule's border is not well-defined or clearly visualized, it is classified as ill-defined and receives zero points. Any margin that cannot be definitively classified as smooth, irregular, or lobulated should be placed into the ill-defined category. Protrusion of the nodule margin into the thyroid capsule is classified as extrathyroid extension (ETE) and warrants an assignment of 3 points.[46,47] Benign nodules are more likely to demonstrate a smooth border, but it should be noted that between 33% and 93% of malignant nodules also present with smooth borders.[47,53,58] Lobulated or irregular margins are thought to

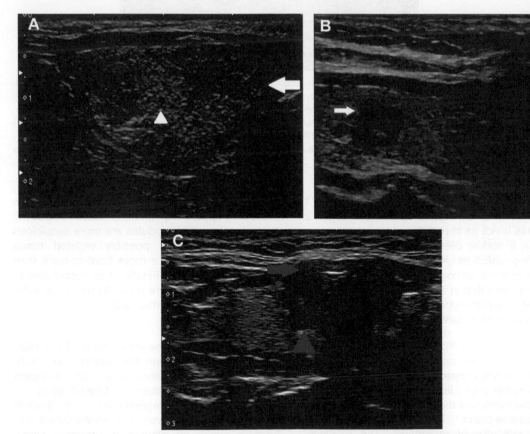

Fig. 13. (*A–C*) Nodule margins. (*A*) Longitudinal section shows a smoothly marginated nodule in the right lobe (TR4) (*white arrow*). Note the echogenic foci in this solid isoechoic nodule (*white arrowhead*). FNA revealed a benign colloid nodule (Bethesda II). (*B*) The longitudinal image shows a solid hypoechoic nodule with essentially squared off, spiculated margins (TR4) (*red/white arrow*). Biopsy revealed a papillary carcinoma (Bethesda 6). (*C*) A 2.2-cm solid hypoechoic nodule that deforms the anterior surface of the thyroid, with possible extrathyroidal extension (TR5) (*red arrow*). Note the markedly lobulated margins (*red arrowhead*). Biopsy revealed a papillary carcinoma (Bethesda 5), which was confirmed at surgery.

represent aggressive growth and thus these features are more suspicious for nodule malignancy.[55] A caveat is that focal areas of thyroiditis can also present with irregular margins. Ill-defined margins have been shown to have no statistically significant association with malignancy and can be seen with benign hyperplastic nodules and focal thyroiditis.[23,53,59]

ETE is characterized by unambiguous invasion into the adjacent soft tissue structures and suggests invasive and more aggressive malignancy (see **Fig. 5**). In the presence of thyroid border contour bulging, loss of the echogenic thyroid border or border abutment, minimal ETE may be suspected. However, caution should be used when classifying a nodule as demonstrating minimal ETE, because agreement among imagers and pathologists of this process is poor and the clinical significance not clear.[46,60–63]

Echogenic foci

A focal region of markedly increased echogenicity relative to the adjacent nodule is the definition of a thyroid nodule echogenic focus (EF).[47] They may be isolated or may present with various types of posterior acoustic artifact and are associated with both malignant and benign lesions.[64] In general, independent of the additional nodule parenchymal features, all categories of EF, save for those with large comet tail artifacts, are associated with an increased risk of thyroid malignancy[49] (**Fig. 14**).

Punctate EF are defined as dotlike foci, being less than 1 mm in size. In the past, all punctate EF within nodules were classified as microcalcifications; however, this term is a misnomer, because not all EF are psammomatous microcalcifications of PTC. These punctate foci may also represent the back wall of tiny cysts or inspissated crystals, such as those seen in colloid nodules. True psammomatous microcalcifications will not exhibit posterior acoustic shadowing given their small size. These true microcalcifications are found in 29% to 59% of all primary thyroid cancers, most commonly PTC.[43,47,49] A comet tail artifact is a form of reverberation artifact between 2 reflective interfaces resulting in closely spaced reflective echoes. On US examination, this artifact manifests as a triangular shape posterior to the EF, owing to the later echoes decreasing in amplitude secondary to attenuation.[49] Traditionally, all EF with comet tail artifacts were thought to be an indicator of benignity; however, studies have shown only those comet tail artifacts larger than 1 mm are almost always benign and associated with colloid, thus receiving a score of 0 points.[49] Conversely, the rate of malignancy in EF

demonstrating a small (<1 mm) comet tail artifacts is similar to those without posterior acoustic artifact. Thus, EF with no posterior artifact or those with small comet tail artifacts receive a score of 3 points.

Macrocalcifications are EF larger than 1 mm with posterior acoustic shadowing. Thought to be secondary to tissue necrosis, these EF are true dysplastic calcifications Approximately 15% of nodules with these course calcifications harbor malignancy; thus, they are assigned 1 point.[49]

Peripheral rim calcifications are those shadowing EF that lie along all or a part of the nodule's border and are also true calcifications. In the literature, these have also been referred to as eggshell or rim calcifications. Some studies have indicated a stronger association of malignancy with this specific type of macrocalcification, thus the 2-point designation in TIRADS.[49,65] Occasionally, shadowing artifact from these macrocalcifications will limit or even preclude assessment of the nodule's internal features, such as composition and echogenicity (**Fig. 15**). In this scenario, it may be prudent to assume the nodule is solid and assign 2 points for composition and, as discussed elsewhere in this article, 1 point for echogenicity.

Finally, punctate EF may be encountered in spongiform nodules, where they most likely represent the back wall of tiny benign cysts. The point total for the spongiform nodule in this case should not be increased, because the EFs in these nodules are not considered suspicious.[43]

Size

Thyroid nodule size is not included in the TIRADS scoring system but does play a role in the follow-up recommendations; no imaging follow-up, US follow-up, or FNAB.[46,47] Specifically, TIRADS is congruent with most other guidelines in only recommending FNAB for suspicious nodules 1 cm in size or larger. Nodule size is not an independent predictor of malignant risk in PTC, thus its exclusion from the scoring system.[46,66,67] Large nodules are often benign and very small nodules may be malignant; nodule characteristics other than size have consistently proven to be a more reliable indicator of a nodule being benign or malignant (**Fig. 16**). Although occult small thyroid cancers are increasing in frequency, they are thought to be of doubtful clinical significance and indolent, solid highly suspicious nodules with features that are too small to warrant FNAB (<1 cm) should nevertheless receive US follow-up to decrease the chance that an eventual clinically significant malignancy will not be overlooked.[43,68,69]

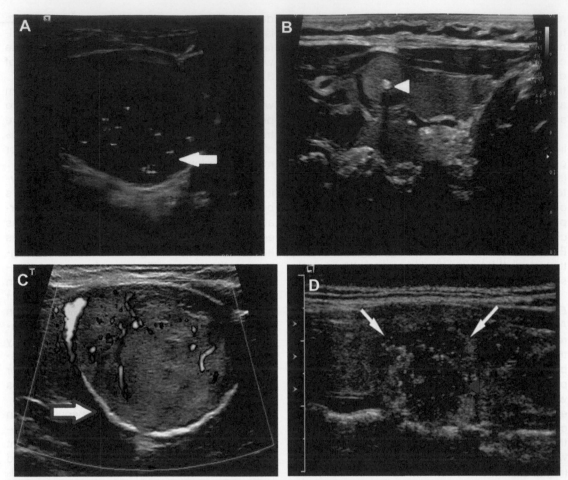

Fig. 14. (*A–D*) Echogenic foci. (*A*) Transverse image shows a large cystic lesion that contains multiple echogenic foci demonstrating large comet tail artifacts (TR1) (*white arrow*). A biopsy was not performed. These are another of the so-called leave alone lesions. Because these are likely colloid, FNA would be compromised by an inability to withdraw diagnostic material. (*B*) A small echogenic nodule with a relatively large shadowing macrocalcification (*white arrowheads*). Although the overall features were consistent with a TR4 lesion, follow-up was undertaken given the small size. The lesion has been stable for 2 years. (*C*) A longitudinal image through the left lobe of the thyroid reveals a peripherally calcified lesion that is internally solid and isoechoic (TR4) (*red/white arrow*). A biopsy was unsuccessful, which is a problem encountered more frequently in peripherally calcified nodules than in other lesions. The surgical specimen revealed a benign follicular nodule. (*D*) Solid nodule found in a 43-year-old woman on a recent MR imaging of the C-spine (*white arrows*). Note the numerous punctate echogenic foci, some of which have small (<1 mm) comet tail artifacts (TR5) (*red arrowhead*). Unlike the large comet tail artifacts shown in Fig. 14A, small comet tails are not considered a sign of benign nodules and are classified along with other punctate echogenic foci. FNA confirmed papillary carcinoma (Bethesda VI).

Additional Considerations

The definition of significant interval enlargement of a thyroid nodule in TIRADS is akin to that used by the American Thyroid Association guidelines; 20% increase in at least 2 nodule dimensions and minimal increase of 2 mm or a 50% increase in nodule volume.[5,47] There is a paucity of consensus in the literature regarding the optimal spacing of follow-up US for nodules that fail to meet the threshold for FNAB because of size. Less than 1 year is not recommended, unless special circumstances such as proven cancers under active surveillance.[70,71] For TR5 lesions, an annual US scan is recommended for up to 5 years. TR4 lesions can be scanned at 1, 2, 3, and 5 years and TR3 lesions scanned at 1, 3, and 5 years. Imaging can stop after the fifth year of follow-up US because nodules showing no significant growth at this time point are considered benign.[46,72] Nodules that exhibit

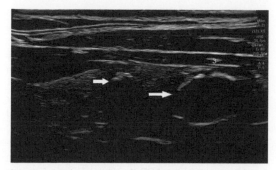

Fig. 15. ensely peripherally calcified nodule. Longitudinal image through right lobe of the thyroid shows 2 nodules with peripheral calcifications that are dense enough to obscure the internal contents making assessment impossible (*white arrows*). According to the TIRADS system, in addition to the 2 points assigned for the peripheral calcifications and 3 points are assigned arbitrarily—2 points for a presumed solid composition and 1 for echogenicity.

interval significant growth but remain below the size threshold for FNAB should be followed with US examination in 1 year.[43,46,47]

It is impractical to biopsy every nodule in glands that present with multiple nodules that are similar in appearance. When multiple nodules are present, the ACR Committee recommends that no

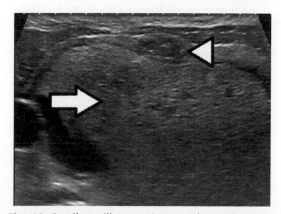

Fig. 16. Small papillary carcinoma. The patient was referred for a biopsy of the large echogenic nodule (*white arrow*). A small solid, hypoechoic nodule with punctate echogenic foci was found incidentally (TR5) (*white arrowhead*). After discussion with the patient, a biopsy was performed and papillary carcinoma diagnosed. Nodule size is not actually taken into consideration as a diagnostic feature in the TIRADS scheme because it has not been shown to be associated with malignancy. It has been included in the decision-making process for biopsy based on association with outcome.

more than 4 nodules receive TIRADS point scores. The 4 most suspicious appearing nodules should be scored. In addition, as mentioned elsewhere in this article, size is not an independent risk factor for malignancy and there is no evidence that performing an FNAB on the largest nodule, regardless of its US appearance, improves patient outcome. For this reason, the usage of such terminology as "dominant nodule" is discouraged. FNAB of only the 2 nodules with the highest point totals is recommended, regardless if multiple nodules are preset.[43,46,47]

FUTURE CONSIDERATIONS AND SUMMARY

The ACR-TIRADS provides a standardized method to aid in the management of thyroid nodules seen on US imaging. However, variability in assigning US features by practitioners using TIRADS will result in inconsistent management. A study in 2018 focusing on TIRADS use demonstrated that interobserver agreement was fair to moderate for all features except shape and macrocalcifications, which had substantial agreement.[73] The results of this study suggest that continued training and education regarding the use of TIRADS is important and necessary. Despite the variability in assigning features, however, the adoption of TIRADS does improve agreement for recommending biopsy overall. Furthermore, applying TIRADS results in a reduced number of thyroid nodules biopsied while also improving the specificity and accuracy in the detection of malignancy.[45,73–75] In addition, the chance of missing a malignancy is greatly diminished because most malignant nodules not recommended for biopsy will, at the very least, receive a recommendation for follow-up US surveillance.

In the future, the application of machine learning and artificial intelligence in the risk stratification of thyroid nodules will likely become prevalent.[76] A study in 2019 concluded that an artificial intelligence–optimized TIRADS system validated the non–machine-assisted TIRADS and slightly improved the specificity of detecting malignant nodules while maintaining sensitivity.[77] Nodule feature assignments were also simplified, an outcome that may eventually improve ease of use.

In summary, the recommendations provided by TIRADS greatly assist in the management of thyroid nodules evaluated with US examination. Compared with other existing guidelines, TIRADS results in a meaningful decrease in the number of thyroid nodules biopsied and significantly improves the specificity of cancer detection without sacrificing sensitivity.

CLINICS CARE POINTS

- Thyroid nodules, whether benign or malignant, are common in the adult population.

- Currently, FNAB is the gold standard technique to determine whether a nodule is malignant or may require surgery to establish definite diagnosis.

- Most thyroid nodules are benign however; thus, not all detected nodules require FNAB.

- US examination has emerged as the optimal noninvasive imaging modality in helping to determine which nodules demonstrate suspicious features of malignancy, and thus warrant further evaluation with FNAB.

- In 2017, the ACR TIRADS committee published a white paper with a standardized (lexicon) approach to classifying nodules on US examination, termed TIRADS.

- The US examination features in TIRADS are categorized as benign, minimally suspicious, moderately suspicious, or highly suspicious for malignancy. Points are given for all the US examination features in a nodule, with more suspicious features being awarded additional points.

- Applying TIRADS results in a meaningful reduction in the number of thyroid nodules biopsied and significantly improves the specificity of cancer detection without sacrificing sensitivity.

DISCLOSURE

No conflicts of interest to disclose.

REFERENCES

1. Ferlay J, Colombet M, Soerjomataram I, et al. Estimating the global cancer incidence and mortality in 2018: GLOBOCAN sources and methods. Int J Cancer 2019;144(8):1941–53.

2. Cancer Fast Stats. National Cancer Institute. Available at: http://seer.cancer.gov/faststats/. Accessed October 25, 2020.

3. Chung R, Kim D. Imaging of thyroid nodules. Appl Radiol 2019;48(1):16–26.

4. Wilhelm S. Evaluation of thyroid incidentaloma. Surg Clin North Am 2014;94(3):485–97.

5. Haugen BR, Alexander EK, Bible KC, et al. 2015 American Thyroid Association management guidelines for adult patients with thyroid nodules and differentiated thyroid cancer: the American Thyroid Association Guidelines task force on thyroid nodules and differentiated thyroid cancer. Thyroid 2016; 26(1):1–133.

6. Grani G, Sponziello M, Pecce V, et al. Contemporary thyroid nodule evaluation and management. J Clin Endocrinol Metab 2020;105(9):2869–83.

7. Ahn HS, Kim HJ, Welch HG. Korea's thyroid-cancer "epidemic"–screening and overdiagnosis. N Engl J Med 2014;371(19):1765–7.

8. Hoang JK, Langer JE, Middleton WD, et al. Managing incidental thyroid nodules detected on imaging: white paper of the ACR Incidental Thyroid Findings Committee. J Am Coll Radiol 2015;12(2):143–50.

9. Moon JH, Hyun MK, Lee JY, et al. Prevalence of thyroid nodules and their associated clinical parameters: a large-scale, multicenter-based health checkup study. Korean J Intern Med 2018;33(4): 753–62.

10. Vaccarella S, Franceschi S, Bray F, et al. Worldwide Thyroid-Cancer Epidemic? The Increasing Impact of Overdiagnosis. N Engl J Med 2016;375(7):614–7.

11. Kitahara CM, Sosa JA. The changing incidence of thyroid cancer. Nat Rev Endocrinol 2016;12(11): 646–53.

12. Dal Maso L, Panato C, Franceschi S, et al. The impact of overdiagnosis on thyroid cancer epidemic in Italy,1998-2012. Eur J Cancer 2018;94:6–15.

13. Shi LL, DeSantis C, Jemal A, et al. Changes in thyroid cancer incidence, post-2009 American Thyroid Association guidelines. Laryngoscope 2017; 127(10):2437–41.

14. Morris LG, Tuttle RM, Davies L. Changing Trends in the Incidence of Thyroid Cancer in the United States. JAMA Otolaryngol Head Neck Surg 2016; 142(7):709–11.

15. Vargas-Uricoechea H, Meza-Cabrera I, Herrera-Chaparro J. Concordance between the TIRADS ultrasound criteria and the BETHESDA cytology criteria on the nontoxic thyroid nodule. Thyroid Res 2017;10:1.

16. Yang J, Schnadig V, Logrono R, et al. Fine-needle aspiration of thyroid nodules: a study of 4703 patients with histologic and clinical correlations. Cancer 2007;111(5):306–15.

17. Cibas ES, Ali SZ. NCI Thyroid FNA State of the Science Conference. The Bethesda System For Reporting Thyroid Cytopathology. Am J Clin Pathol 2009; 132(5):658–65.

18. Ali SZ, Cibas ES. The Bethesda System for Reporting Thyroid Cytopathology II. Acta Cytol 2016; 60(5):397–8.

19. Langer JE, Baloch ZW, McGrath C, et al. Thyroid nodule fine-needle aspiration. Semin Ultrasound CT MR 2012;33(2):158–65.

20. Nachiappan AC, Metwalli ZA, Hailey BS, et al. The thyroid: review of imaging features and biopsy techniques with radiologic-pathologic correlation.

Radiographics 2014;34(2):276–93 [published correction appears in Radiographics. 2014 Sep-Oct;34(5):8A].

21. Shih ML, Lee JA, Hsieh CB, et al. Thyroidectomy for Hashimoto's thyroiditis: complications and associated cancers. Thyroid 2008;18(7):729–34.

22. Sacks W, Braunstein GD. Papillary thyroid carcinoma. In: Braunstein G, editor. Thyroid cancer. endocrine updates, vol. 32. Boston (MA): Springer; 2015. p. 133–53. Accessed October 27,2020.

23. Hoang JK, Lee WK, Lee M, et al. US Features of thyroid malignancy: pearls and pitfalls. Radiographics 2007;27(3):847–65.

24. Ito Y, Hirokawa M, Higashiyama T, et al. Prognosis and prognostic factors of follicular carcinoma in Japan; importance of postoperative pathological examination. World J Surg 2007;31(7):1417–24.

25. Sanders LE, Silverman M. Follicular and Hürthle cell carcinoma: predicting outcome and directing therapy. Surgery 1998;124(6):967–74.

26. Sillery JC, Reading CC, Charboneau JW, et al. Thyroid follicular carcinoma: sonographic features of 50 cases. AJR Am J Roentgenol 2010;194(1):44–54.

27. Cupisti K, Wolf A, Raffel A, et al. Long term clinical and biochemical follow-up in medullary thyroid carcinoma: a single institution's experience over 20 years. Ann Surg 2007;246(5):815–21.

28. Lee S, Shin JH, Han BK, et al. Medullary thyroid carcinoma: comparison with papillary thyroid carcinoma and application of current sonographic criteria. AJR Am J Roentgenol 2010;194(4):1090–4.

29. Ganeshan D, Paulson E, Duran C, et al. Current update on medullary thyroid carcinoma. AJR Am J Roentgenol 2013;201(6):W867–76.

30. Aldinger KA, Samaan NA, Ibanez M, et al. Anaplastic carcinoma of the thyroid: a review of 84 cases of spindle and giant cell carcinoma of the thyroid. Cancer 1978;41(6):2267–75.

31. Hahn SY, Shin JH. Description and Comparison of the Sonographic Characteristics of Poorly Differentiated Thyroid Carcinoma and Anaplastic Thyroid Carcinoma. J Ultrasound Med 2016;35(9):1873–9.

32. Ishikawa H, Tamaki Y, Takahashi M, et al. Comparison of primary thyroid lymphoma with anaplastic thyroid carcinoma on computed tomographic imaging. Radiat Med 2002;20(1):9–15.

33. Ahmed S, Ghazarian MP, Cabanillas ME, et al. Imaging of Anaplastic Thyroid Carcinoma. AJNR Am J Neuroradiol 2018;39(3):547–51.

34. Poppe K, Lahoutte T, Everaert H, et al. The utility of multimodality imaging in anaplastic thyroid carcinoma. Thyroid 2004;14(11):981–2.

35. Takashima S, Morimoto S, Ikezoe J, et al. CT evaluation of anaplastic thyroid carcinoma. AJR Am J Roentgenol 1990;154(5):1079–85.

36. Sharma A, Jasim S, Reading CC, et al. Clinical presentation and diagnostic challenges of thyroid lymphoma: a cohort study. Thyroid 2016;26(8):1061–7.

37. Travaglino A, Pace M, Varricchio S, et al. Hashimoto thyroiditis in primary thyroid non-Hodgkin lymphoma. Am J Clin Pathol 2020;153(2):156–64.

38. Ma B, Jia Y, Wang Q, et al. Ultrasound of primary thyroid non-Hodgkin's lymphoma. Clin Imaging 2014;38(5):621–6.

39. Xia Y, Wang L, Jiang Y, et al. Sonographic appearance of primary thyroid lymphoma-preliminary experience. PLoS One 2014;9(12):e114080.

40. HooKim K, Gaitor J, Lin O, et al. Secondary tumors involving the thyroid gland: A multi-institutional analysis of 28 cases diagnosed on fine-needle aspiration. Diagn Cytopathol 2015;43(11):904–11.

41. Pastorello RG, Saieg MA. Metastases to the thyroid: potential cytologic mimics of primary thyroid neoplasms. Arch Pathol Lab Med 2019;143(3):394–9.

42. Hegedüs L. Thyroid ultrasound. Endocrinol Metab Clin North Am 2001;30(2):339–ix.

43. Tessler FN, Middleton WD, Grant EG. Thyroid Imaging Reporting and Data System (TI-RADS): a user's guide. Radiology 2018;287(1):29–36 [published correction appears in Radiology. 2018 Jun;287(3):1082].

44. Ha EJ, Na DG, Baek JH, et al. US fine-needle aspiration biopsy for thyroid malignancy: diagnostic performance of seven society guidelines applied to 2000 thyroid nodules. Radiology 2018;287(3):893–900.

45. Middleton WD, Teefey SA, Reading CC, et al. Comparison of Performance Characteristics of American College of Radiology TI-RADS, Korean Society of Thyroid Radiology TIRADS, and American Thyroid Association Guidelines. AJR Am J Roentgenol 2018;210(5):1148–54.

46. Tessler FN, Middleton WD, Grant EG, et al. ACR Thyroid Imaging, Reporting and Data System (TI-RADS): white paper of the ACR TI-RADS committee. J Am Coll Radiol 2017;14(5):587–95.

47. Grant EG, Tessler FN, Hoang JK, et al. Thyroid ultrasound reporting lexicon: white paper of the ACR Thyroid Imaging, Reporting and Data System (TI-RADS) Committee. J Am Coll Radiol 2015;12(12 Pt A):1272–9.

48. Frates MC, Benson CB, Charboneau JW, et al. Management of thyroid nodules detected at US: Society of Radiologists in Ultrasound consensus conference statement. Radiology 2005;237(3):794–800.

49. Malhi H, Beland MD, Cen SY, et al. Echogenic foci in thyroid nodules: significance of posterior acoustic artifacts. AJR Am J Roentgenol 2014;203(6):1310–6.

50. Moon HJ, Kwak JY, Kim MJ, et al. Can vascularity at power Doppler US help predict thyroid malignancy? Radiology 2010;255(1):260–9.

51. Rosario PW, Silva AL, Borges MA, et al. Is Doppler ultrasound of additional value to gray-scale

ultrasound in differentiating malignant and benign thyroid nodules? Arch Endocrinol Metab 2015; 59(1):79–83.

52. Frates MC, Benson CB, Doubilet PM, et al. Prevalence and distribution of carcinoma in patients with solitary and multiple thyroid nodules on sonography. J Clin Endocrinol Metab 2006;91(9):3411–7.

53. Moon WJ, Jung SL, Lee JH, et al. Benign and malignant thyroid nodules: US differentiation–multicenter retrospective study. Radiology 2008;247(3):762–70.

54. Moon HJ, Kwak JY, Kim EK, et al. A taller-than-wide shape in thyroid nodules in transverse and longitudinal ultrasonographic planes and the prediction of malignancy. Thyroid 2011;21(11):1249–53.

55. Kim EK, Park CS, Chung WY, et al. New sonographic criteria for recommending fine-needle aspiration biopsy of nonpalpable solid nodules of the thyroid. AJR Am J Roentgenol 2002;178(3):687–91.

56. Kwak JY, Han KH, Yoon JH, et al. Thyroid imaging reporting and data system for US features of nodules: a step in establishing better stratification of cancer risk. Radiology 2011;260(3):892–9.

57. Na DG, Baek JH, Sung JY, et al. Thyroid imaging reporting and data system risk stratification of thyroid nodules: categorization based on solidity and echogenicity. Thyroid 2016;26(4):562–72.

58. Ahn SS, Kim EK, Kang DR, et al. Biopsy of thyroid nodules: comparison of three sets of guidelines. AJR Am J Roentgenol 2010;194(1):31–7.

59. Chan BK, Desser TS, McDougall IR, et al. Common and uncommon sonographic features of papillary thyroid carcinoma. J Ultrasound Med 2003;22(10): 1083–90.

60. Shin JH, Ha TK, Park HK, et al. Implication of minimal extrathyroidal extension as a prognostic factor in papillary thyroid carcinoma. Int J Surg 2013; 11(9):944–7.

61. Su HK, Wenig BM, Haser GC, et al. Inter-observer variation in the pathologic identification of minimal extrathyroidal extension in papillary thyroid carcinoma. Thyroid 2016;26(4):512–7.

62. Kwak JY, Kim EK, Youk JH, et al. Extrathyroid extension of well-differentiated papillary thyroid microcarcinoma on US. Thyroid 2008;18(6):609–14.

63. Kamaya A, Tahvildari AM, Patel BN, et al. Sonographic detection of extracapsular extension in papillary thyroid cancer. J Ultrasound Med 2015; 34(12):2225–30.

64. Lacout A, Chevenet C, Thariat J, et al. Thyroid calcifications: a pictorial essay. J Clin Ultrasound 2016; 44(4):245–51.

65. Arpaci D, Ozdemir D, Cuhaci N, et al. Evaluation of cytopathological findings in thyroid nodules with macrocalcification: macrocalcification is not innocent as it seems. Arq Bras Endocrinol Metabol 2014;58(9):939–45.

66. Jinih M, Faisal F, Abdalla K, et al. Association between thyroid nodule size and malignancy rate. Ann R Coll Surg Engl 2020;102(1):43–8.

67. Hong MJ, Na DG, Baek JH, et al. Impact of Nodule Size on Malignancy Risk Differs according to the Ultrasonography Pattern of Thyroid Nodules. Korean J Radiol 2018;19(3):534–41.

68. Ito Y, Miyauchi A, Inoue H, et al. An observational trial for papillary thyroid microcarcinoma in Japanese patients. World J Surg 2010;34(1):28–35.

69. Davies L, Roman BR, Fukushima M, et al. Patient Experience of Thyroid Cancer Active Surveillance in Japan. JAMA Otolaryngol Head Neck Surg 2019;145(4):363–70.

70. Ajmal S, Rapoport S, Ramirez Batlle H, et al. The natural history of the benign thyroid nodule: what is the appropriate follow-up strategy? J Am Coll Surg 2015;220(6):987–92.

71. Nakamura H, Hirokawa M, Ota H, et al. Is an Increase in Thyroid Nodule Volume a Risk Factor for Malignancy? Thyroid 2015;25(7):804–11.

72. Durante C, Costante G, Lucisano G, et al. The natural history of benign thyroid nodules. JAMA 2015; 313(9):926–35.

73. Hoang JK, Middleton WD, Farjat AE, et al. Interobserver Variability of Sonographic Features Used in the American College of Radiology Thyroid Imaging Reporting and Data System. AJR Am J Roentgenol 2018;211(1):162–7.

74. Grani G, Lamartina L, Ascoli V, et al. Reducing the number of unnecessary thyroid biopsies while improving diagnostic accuracy: toward the "right" TI-RADS. J Clin Endocrinol Metab 2019;104(1):95–102.

75. Wu XL, Du JR, Wang H, et al. Comparison and preliminary discussion of the reasons for the differences in diagnostic performance and unnecessary FNA biopsies between the ACR TIRADS and 2015 ATA guidelines. Endocrine 2019;65(1):121–31.

76. Buda M, Wildman-Tobriner B, Hoang JK, et al. Management of thyroid nodules seen on US images: deep learning may match performance of radiologists. Radiology 2019;292(3):695–701.

77. Wildman-Tobriner B, Buda M, Hoang JK, et al. Using artificial intelligence to revise ACR TI-RADS risk stratification of thyroid nodules: diagnostic accuracy and utility. Radiology 2019;292(1):112–9.

Preoperative Molecular Testing of Thyroid Nodules
Current Concepts

Michelle D. Williams, MD

KEYWORDS

- Molecular testing • Indeterminate thyroid nodules • Fine needle aspiration

KEY POINTS

- Molecular assessment is commercially available for further evaluation of cytologically indeterminate thyroid nodules to aid in surgical triage based on risk level of malignancy.
- Testing performance including positive and negative predictive values will vary based on the prevalence of thyroid cancer in the population being evaluated.
- Improved assays have enhanced classification of indeterminate Hurthle cell nodules.
- Testing methodology and performance are important considerations in determining when a patient may be monitored following testing.
- Testing results should not negate clinical risk factors indicating surgical resection.

BACKGROUND

Molecular assessment in thyroid nodules began with the search for ancillary tools to aid the triage of patients with indeterminate thyroid nodules by fine needle aspiration (FNA) cytologic assessment. Of the 15% to 30% of indeterminate nodules, approximately 75% will be benign following surgical resection required for definitive classification.[1,2] Through enhanced understanding of molecular alterations associated with thyroid tumorigenesis, multiple commercially available assays are now available in the CLIA (Clinical Laboratory Improved Amendments)-approved setting for evaluating cytologically indeterminate thyroid nodules.[3–5] Moreover, the expansion of these assays continues to enhance testing performance.[6–8] Molecular diagnostic advancement in thyroid nodule assessment has also benefited from the combined skills of clinicians acquiring ultrasound-guided targeted tissue samples via FNA biopsy and the associated development of molecular techniques that can reliably assess alterations using nanograms of material.[9] The results are clinically validated platforms enabling enhanced evaluation in the preoperative setting for cytologically indeterminate thyroid nodules. These testing results allow a subset of patients to be monitored without surgical intervention similarly to a benign FNA and for others increasing the pretest probability of malignancy base on molecular alterations detected. The American Thyroid Association, European Thyroid Association, as well as the National Comprehensive Cancer Network (NCCN) and others mention molecular testing and how it may be integrated into thyroid nodule evaluation.[10–14] However, challenges still remain as to who to test, uncertainties of long-term testing outcomes, and the recognition that ancillary molecular testing may not play a role if other clinical factors warrant surgery.

CYTOLOGICALLY INDETERMINATE THYROID NODULES

A refined thyroid FNA classification known as the Bethesda System for Reporting Thyroid Cytopathology allows for clinical triage of up to 80% of patients based on cytologic findings (**Table 1**).[1,15,16] The remaining nodules are

Department of Pathology, University of Texas MD Anderson Cancer Center, 1515 Holcombe Boulevard, Unit 085, Houston, TX 77030, USA
E-mail address: mdwillia@mdanderson.org

Neuroimag Clin N Am 31 (2021) 301–312
https://doi.org/10.1016/j.nic.2021.04.009
1052-5149/21/© 2021 Elsevier Inc. All rights reserved.

Table 1
The Bethesda system for reporting thyroid cytopathology and associated risk of malignancy[1,15,16]

Bethesda Diagnostic Category I-VI. and Corresponding Cytologic Diagnosis	Frequency of Each Diagnostic Category (%) (Range) Meta-Analysis 25,445 FNAs[1]	% Malignancy by Bethesda Range vs (% Found in the Meta-Analysis 6362 Surgeries[1]	Clinical Triage	Molecular Consideration[10]
I. Nondiagnostic "inadequate"	13 (2–24)	1–4 (16)	Repeat aspiration with ultrasound (best strategy)	Low-yield
II. Benign	59 (39–74)	0–3 (3.7)	Observation	Not recommended
III. aAtypia of undetermined significance or follicular lesion of undetermined significance (AUS/FLUS)	10 (3–27)	5–15 (16)	In conjunction with radiographic & clinical factors: • Repeat FNA (AUS/FLUS)	Molecular assessment to rule-in or rule out malignancy based on testing performance
IV. aFollicular neoplasm or suspicious for follicular neoplasm (FN/SFN)	10 (1–25)	15–30 (26)	• Repeat ultrasound evaluation @6–12 mo (AUS/FLUS) vs • Surgery vs molecular (FN/SFN)	
V. Suspicious for malignancy	3 (1–6)	60–75 (75)	Surgical resection	Molecular rule in type testing may aid in surgical decision making[b]
VI. Malignant	5 (2–16)	97–99 (98.6)	Surgical resection	Not recommended for diagnosis

Abbreviation: FNA, fine needle aspiration.

[a] Indeterminate categories.

[b] Note: negative testing cannot negate a cytologically suspicious FNA diagnosis; The presence of certain mutations or combination of mutations may aid in risk stratification for local recurrence and discussions regarding initial surgical planning.[34]

"indeterminate" with 10% of thyroid FNAs falling into cytologic diagnostic category III, Atypia of undetermined significance or follicular lesion of undetermined significance (AUS/FLUS) and similarly, 10% into category IV, Follicular neoplasm or suspicious for follicular neoplasm (FN/SFN). The differential diagnosis of indeterminate thyroid nodules includes benign and malignant entities including cellular adenomatous change, follicular adenomas, follicular carcinomas, and follicular variant of papillary thyroid carcinoma and noninvasive follicular thyroid neoplasms with papillary like nuclei (NIFTP). Cytologic features of indeterminate FNA cannot determine benign from malignant as architectural features, specifically capsular and or lymphovascular invasion are used to define malignancy.[17–19] It is also important to recognize that the risk for malignancy in each Bethesda category is dependent on the cytopathology and cancer prevalence in the population being evaluated.[15] American Thyroid Association (ATA) guidelines highlight that although a risk of malignancy is noted in the Bethesda classification book for each category, the risk of malignancy will vary by institution and should be defined locally to help choose appropriate molecular testing and interpret the testing performance.[10]

Molecular Considerations

Current molecular assessments available for thyroid nodules arose from 2 different principals: testing that can "rule out" malignancy with high specificity and negative predictive value versus a test that "rules in" malignancy and neoplasms for which surgery would be warranted. Testing evolution has expanded platforms with both of these goals. It is also important to recognize that sensitivity and specificity are parameters based on test performance; however, negative and positive predicative values as reported in studies will vary when translated to a different population based on the prevalence of malignancy (**Fig. 1**). Understanding the testing performance in these 2 distinct testing approaches and how they translate to a patient's risk of malignancy and application in surgical triage is essential in counseling patients.

RULE OUT testing
The initial efforts to decrease unnecessary surgery in patients with ultimately benign nodules led to the development of a gene expression assay focused on developing a highly sensitive test with a robust negative predictive value to mirror the negative cytologic malignancy rate of ∼ 4%. The initial gene expression classifier (GEC) assay used 167 gene expression levels (messenger

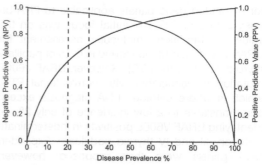

Fig. 1. Influence of disease prevalence on PPVs and NPVs. Mock example of receiver operator curves of a test's performance. Specifically the NPV and PPV will vary based on the disease prevalence in the population being tested. In a population with a 20% disease prevalence, there is a higher NPV compared with a population with a 30% disease prevalence. The PPV also varies and will be higher in the population with higher disease prevalence.

RNA [mRNA]) to classify indeterminate FNA cytologic samples into "benign" or "suspicious."[20] This assay required centralized pathology read of the FNA slides to overcome adherent challenges that arise within the pathologic classification of thyroid FNA biopsies. If the thyroid FNA biopsy was diagnosed as an indeterminate Bethesda classification, then the GEC assay was performed. The validation study was a prospective, multicenter study of 577 cytologically indeterminate thyroid aspirates with 413 pathologically examined nodules by surgery.[20] The GEC initial performance showed a negative predictive value of 95% and 94% in indeterminate Bethesda category III and IV respectively. Sensitivity to accurately classify malignancies was 90% with a modest specificity of 52% in identifying benign nodules in Bethesda category III or IV indeterminate thyroid nodules. The initial studies also included testing suspicious nodules (Bethesda category V) to try to identify the subset in that category (∼ 25%) without malignancy; however, the testing performance was insufficient to continue recommending the practice of GEC in suspicious nodules. Additional independent institutional studies were subsequently reported for which disease prevalence was highlighted as critical to testing performance.[12,21,22]

RULE IN testing
A testing method with high specificity and positive predictive value are desired for an assay for disease detection. The combination of detailed genomic knowledge in thyroid carcinogenesis through The Cancer Genome Atlas (TCGA) and other investigations along with advancements in next-generation sequencing technologies allowed

for expanded gene panels applicable to FNA biopsy samples.[23–25] The initial focus was on the value of standalone molecular assessment for BRAF V600E, a mutation found in 60% of papillary thyroid carcinomas (PTC). However, BRAF V600E mutation is associated with conventional PTC, which is where cytology FNA diagnosis excels. This translates to a low incidence of only 2% of identifying BRAF V600E positivity in indeterminate Category III and IV thyroid nodules.[26] Expanded DNA panels were then proposed; however, without including fusion genes in the evaluation, the assay will inherently underperform in sensitivity. Fusions are the main oncogenic event in a subset of thyroid cancers including follicular carcinoma and PTC.[27] TCGA found 15% fusions in the 496 PTCs occurring in both conventional and the follicular variant.[23] Fusions also occur in follicular adenoma, follicular carcinomas, and NIFTP, all of which fall into indeterminate thyroid cytology.[27] Molecular assessment for gene fusions remains challenging often requiring assays for each gene, the multiple potential breakpoints and gene partners for detection. Methodologies often require mRNA, which is labile compared with DNA. As novel fusion partners are still being reported, testing continues to evolve to further coverage the spectrum of fusions now associated with thyroid malignancies.

A minimum of a 7 gene panel including fusions (BRAF, HRAS, NRAS, KRAS, and RET/PTC1, RET/PTC3 and PAX8/PPARG fusions) provides a starting point for thyroid-specific molecular assessment. These combined gene alterations have a sensitivity of 48% to 81% in detecting malignancy in indeterminate nodules across multiple platforms and institutions.[28,29] Thus, this limited panel as a rule-in test when positive signifies a higher risk of malignancy (Table 2); however, the test is not sensitive enough to exclude malignancy when reported as negative for alterations. To enhance testing performance, specifically sensitivity, further expansion to incorporate new alterations and gene fusions associated with thyroid cancer were added. Further expansion of next-generation sequencing (NGS) assays followed with provided proof of concept in thyroid FNA, frozen and formalin-fixed paraffin-embedded samples followed by a formal assay Thyroseq, which evaluated 12 genes for 284 mutational hot spots, using only 5 to 10 ng of DNA.[30] The resulting iterations led to expansion of genes concurrently evaluated for evolving from a 7-gene panel (2007) and 15-gene panel (Thyroseq) (2013), to Thyroseq v2 a 56-gene panel (2014) and the current clinically offered Thyroseq v3 evaluating a 112-gene panel.[8,28,30,31] With these expanded

Table 2
Risk of malignancy based on genes altered in thyroid malignancies[8,33–35]

Molecular Alterations with High Probability of Malignancy >95–99%	
Mutations	**Fusions**
BRAFV600E[a,b]	RET/PTC[a]
P53	NTRK[a]
TERTp	
RET	

Molecular Alterations with Intermediate Risk of Malignancy 40%–60%	
Mutations	**Fusions**
BRAF K601E	PPARgamma[a]
RAS (N > H > K)[a]	Thada
EIF1AX	
PTEN	

[a] Included in the minimal panel to consider for indeterminate thyroid nodule testing.
[b] False positive testing has been reported at 1:1000.

panels, the sensitivity improved from 60% to 90% then 94%.[32] Note that these values vary slightly by Bethesda III versus IV categories and are lower in Hurthle cell rich nodules as discussed later in this article.

In Rule-in molecular testing, the presence of a molecular alteration increases the probability of a thyroid malignancy in nodules identified as intermediate to high-risk based on the type of alteration identified. This in turn assists with the clinical discussion and triage to surgery for diagnosis and treatment. **Table 2** highlights that some molecular alterations are oncogenic and synonymous with malignancy, such as BRAF V600E (>98% risk),[33] whereas other mutations, including RAS, are thought to occur early in tumorigenesis and are seen in the spectrum of thyroid neoplasms from adenomas through carcinomas. The pretest probability of cancer is approximately 40% to 60% risk of malignancy when a RAS mutation is detected.[8,33–35] However as more data are accumulated, there is further validation and potential information at the specific variant level. In a meta-analysis of thyroid FNA, the positive predictive value (PPV) by specific mutation was 63% for HRAS versus 38% for NRAS and 25% for KRAS; however, it is critical to know and may not have been able to be determined how NIFTP was counted in these studies.[33] As these intermediate-risk mutations evaluated in these panels are viewed as pre-neoplastic, triage to diagnostic lobectomy should be considered when identified. However, continued clinical correlation and counseling of the meaning of molecular alterations related to the specific gene(s) involved is necessary.

False positive mutational testing can occur, although is rare and will be platform specific. Thyroseq noted false positive BRAF V600E in 1:1000 test results. Other causes of false negative results include low level of tumor to background cells in a cytologic sample (below threshold for detection) and sampling issues. Malignancy may also be identified with negative testing, as a small subset of thyroid carcinomas still remain without known driver mutation or gene fusion.

EXPANDED MOLECULAR APPROACHES

For reference, the preceding literature through Thyroseq2 was available at the time the ATA 2015 and the 2017 European guidances were developed, which are detailed later in this article.[10,12] It is critical to acknowledge this breakpoint, as subsequent testing modifications with enhanced performance to be discussed will likely lead to refined guidance in future iterations. As testing identified the strength and potential limitations of each platform, expansion and combination testing was added for enhanced performance. "Rule-out" testing methodologies have crossed over to add "Rule-in" testing mutational assessments and vice versa. Specifically, to improve GEC testing performance, "rule-out testing methodology" was expanded to a Genomic Sequencing Classifier (GSC) adding measurements of genomic copy number, mitochondrial RNA, and modified bioinformatics for risk stratification.[6] On validation studies of 191 indeterminate thyroid nodules, the GSC showed enhanced performance with a sensitivity of 91% and a specificity of 68%.[6] Modifications added were also to refine algorithms for Hurthle cell rich FNA assessment as discussed further later in this article. Furthermore, for thyroid nodules found to be suspicious by GSC, an additional platform Xpression Atlas screens the RNA for 235 fusions and 905 DNA variants in 593 genes associated with thyroid cancer. This additional level of detail may allow for further risk stratification by molecular variant.[33]

Another novel approach integrates microRNA (miRNA) assessment into thyroid nodule evaluations.[7,36,37] miRNA is single-stranded noncoding RNA strands around 22 nucleotides that play a role in posttranscriptional gene expression. Using a 10 miRNA GEC for stratification, mutational negative thyroid nodules are further classified into positive (malignant) or negative (benign). Risk stratification by miRNA (ThyraMIR) has shown

a high negative predictive value (NPV) and high PPV when combined with a mutation panel test (ThyGenX) of 94% (NPV) with a 32% cancer prevalence in initial studies.[7,37] Further validation of this combined approached termed MPTX on 197 nodules highlights continued high sensitivity (95%) and 90% specificity in Bethesda Category III and IV thyroid nodules by cytology.[37] This study also added a moderate risk group for reporting aligning with Ras or Ras-like mutations, which was associated with a ~39% risk of malignant disease.

Current Guidances

Summation of clinical guidances for ATA, European Thyroid Association (ETA), NCCN, and collectively from the American Association of Clinical Endocrinologists (AACE), American College of Endocrinology (ACE), and Associazione Medici Endocrinologi (AME) are highlighted in Box 1.[10,12–14] It is important to note that these commercially available assays have continued to evolve and enhance their testing performance since these guidances were established with the latest versions listed in Table 3. In addition, clinical and radiographic correlations must be considered for each individual when determining how and when to use molecular testing. Long-term follow-up of patients with molecularly classified negative thyroid nodules who have not undergone surgery is still needed.

American Thyroid Association

The 2015 ATA management guidelines for patients with thyroid nodules and differentiated thyroid cancer describes ancillary molecular testing including rule in and rule out approaches for FNA samples to enhance the initial evaluation of thyroid nodules, and highlights the need to counsel patients on the uncertainty of long-term outcomes.[10] The ATA guidance also emphasizes the need for performing molecular testing in a regulated setting to ensure reproducibility of testing. Similarly the performance of such tests should perform similar to the respective cytologic classifications such that rule-out testing result of "benign" should have a risk of malignancy ≤4% similar to Bethesda Category II benign. Recommendations for considering molecular testing vary slightly between Bethesda category III and IV classified thyroid nodules and does extend to consider evaluation in category V, which is still debated across societies and clinicians. Specifically, the use of molecular assessment in the suspicious category may be considered when additional information may inform the extent of surgery (lobectomy vs total thyroidectomy). Caution should be used in

Box 1
Guidelines with recommendations regarding molecular assessment for thyroid nodules[b]

American Thyroid Association (ATA) (2015)

Well-differentiated thyroid cancers and thyroid nodules[10]

- Molecular testing if clinically used should be performed in Clinical Laboratory Improved Amendments (CLIA)/CAP-certified or international equivalent
- Pretest probability of malignancy must be considered when evaluating molecular testing
- Counsel patients regarding potential benefits, limitations, and uncertainties regarding molecular testing

    Category-specific recommendations

        Category I. Inadequate

- Best strategy is repeat FNA
- Molecular testing may be considered although malignancy prevalence is low resulting in low diagnostic yield

        Category III. AUS/FLUS

- Repeat FNA or consider molecular testing
- Surveillance or surgery for inconclusive molecular results

        Category IV. FN/SFN

- Surgery or consider molecular testing; if inconclusive perform diagnostic surgery

        Category V. Suspicious

- Surgery possible mutational panel[c]

        Category VI. Malignant

- Molecular testing is not recommended for diagnosis

Pediatric[11]

- Studies have not validated utility in pediatric population
- Limited studies from single institutional experience[20,38,39]
- Mutational testing, specifically translocations are common (17%)

    ○ When present are highly indicative of malignancy; however, cytologically AUS/FLUS in pediatric population guidance recommends surgical removal even if mutational testing is negative

European Thyroid Association (2017)

Guidelines regarding thyroid nodule molecular FNA cytology diagnostics[12]

    Mutational Panel (7+ alterations)[a]

- Consider for cytologically indeterminate nodules

    GEC currently not recommended for clinical routine use at this time[b]

- Sites the lack of long-term follow-up data on nonsurgical group based on negative GEC
- And variable results in independent studies for PPV, NPV, sensitivity, and specificity

    Category V. Suspicious

- Surgical extent possibly based on mutational panel[c]

The National Comprehensive Cancer Network (NCCN) (thyroid 2020)[13]

Notes the choice of the precise molecular test depends on the cytology and the clinical question being asked. For molecular testing of indeterminate thyroid nodules only if the testing in combination with radiograph performs similar to that risk seen in benign FNA cytology, should observation be considered (approximately <5%)

AACE, ACE, and AME (2016)

Medical Guidelines for the Diagnosis and Management of Thyroid nodules[14]

Molecular Testing

- Should be performed only when results will influence clinical management
- Is not recommended for benign or cytologically malignant thyroid nodules
- Does not replace cytologic interpretation
- A limited gene panel may be considered
- Close follow-up is still recommended for nodules with "negative" molecular testing

No recommendation for or against

- GEC secondary to limited follow-up
- Whether molecular results should alter surgical extent

Abbreviations: AACE, American Association of Clinical Endocrinologists; ACE, American College of Endocrinology; AME, Associazione Medici Endocrinologi; AUS, atypia of undetermined significance; CAP, College of American Pathologists; FLUS, follicular lesion of undetermined significance; FN, follicular neoplasm; FNA, fine needle aspiration; GEC, gene expression classifier; NPV, negative predictive value; PPV, positive predictive value; SFN, suspicious for follicular neoplasm.

[a]Including as a minimum panel of genes (BRAF, NRAS, HRAS, KRAS) and fusions (RET/PTC NTRK, and PAX8/PPARG).

[b]Note: Guidances were written before the updated molecular assessments of GEC to Genomic Sequencing Classifier and updated/most recent version thyroseq3 for improved testing performance in Hurthle-rich samples that may alter future recommendations.

[c]A negative molecular assessment cannot exclude malignancy in Category V and is only used for risk stratification and consideration for surgical extent.

translating molecular findings to extend surgery without a confirmatory diagnosis, as molecular alterations may be encountered in some benign entities and false positive testing may rarely occur. In addition, as the rate of malignancy in the Bethesda Category V is high, a negative mutational assessment does not negate the risk identified by cytologic evaluation.

Validation of molecular testing in pediatric thyroid nodules is still limited.[11,20,38,39] In addition, as this population has a higher percentage of fusion-associated tumors, the composition of testing and sensitivity must be considered. In a series of 15 pediatric thyroid malignancies tested by the 7-gene panel, 60% showed a positive molecular alteration. Using the expanded Thyroseq2 panel, novel fusions were detected in 4 of the 6 remaining originally mutational negative tumors by the 7-gene platform.[40] These findings highlight the need to align testing methodology with populations and tumor-specific features in that population.

European Thyroid Association guidelines
The ETA 2017 guidelines highlights caution in the utility of testing modalities citing limited follow-up studies and variability across studies.[12] Current

recommendation notes a limited mutational panel including BRAF and RAS mutations, and RET/PTC, NTRK and PAX8/PPARG fusions may be considered for cytologically indeterminate thyroid nodule further evaluation. Moreover, as noted in **Table 2**, a conservative surgical approach of lobectomy should be considered in alterations like RAS with secondary overlap between benign and malignant thyroid nodules. In addition, these limited panels cannot exclude malignancy. Larger NGS panels are not advocated at this time nor are other methodologies GEC or miRNA, citing further independent correlative studies and increased follow-up data are needed to have sufficient evidence for clinical recommendations.

The National Comprehensive Cancer Network
The NCCN Guidelines in the evaluation of thyroid nodules is based on Bethesda Categories and includes the consideration for molecular testing for indeterminate nodules.[13] Importantly, NCCN raises the clinical concern of halting further diagnostic workup of indeterminate nodules if the molecular testing is not robust and that the clinical, radiographic, and cytologic factors must also be considered.

Table 3
Commercially available testing methods in thyroid nodule assessment by cytologic classification

Company Alphabetically and Hurthle Performance	No. Indeterminate FNAs (Prevalence of Cancer)	Sensitivity Specificity	NPV PPV	Evaluations	Samples for Testing[c]
Afirma[a]GSC + Afirma Xpression Atlas (XA)[51]	210 (24%)	91% 68%	96% 47%	Genomic Sequencing Classifier (GSC) and expression ATLAS (XA) 594 genes and 235 fusions	• 2 dedicated FNA passes
Hurthle neoplasms[6]		89% 59%			
ThyGenX/ThyraMIR[b][7,36] (MPTX)	178 (30%)	95% 90%	97% 79%	Multiplatform test (MPTX) Next-generation sequencing for 10 gene mutations/DNA + 10 fusions genes/mRNA; Expression analysis 10 miRNA	• 1 dedicated FNA Pass, or • Cell block, or • Cellular diagnostic cytology slides
Hurthle neoplasms[7]	41 (20%)	75% 67%	92% 35%		
ThyroSeq v3[b,44]	247 (28%)	94% 82%	97% 66%	Next-generation sequencing for DNA and RNA: 112 genes including mutations, insertions and deletions, >120 gene fusions, gene expression and copy number alterations	• 1 dedicated FNA Pass or • 2 drops of 1st FNA pass, or • Cell block, or • Cellular diagnostic cytology slides
Hurthle neoplasms[8]	68(62%)	93% 69%	83% 86%		

Abbreviations: FNA, fine needle aspiration; miRNA, microRNA; mRNA, messenger RNA.

[a] Requires central cytopathology review before running a sample except for running a sample except from preauthorized academic centers.

[b] Accepts samples for testing based on the local or central cytologic pathologic diagnosis of an indeterminate Bethesda Category III or IV.

[c] Sample collection kits are provided for each company. As continual updates are expected, please see the corresponding websites for current sample submissions and testing performance.[3-5]

American Association of Clinical Endocrinologists, American College of Endocrinology, and Associazione Medici Endocrinologi

Similarly, the 2016 collaboration among endocrine societies listed here provides principles for what molecular testing can and cannot do.[14] Caution is also noted around implementation of rule-out testing with data still maturing around long-term follow-up particularly when trying to triage patients to observation (rule-out testing). See **Box 1** for overarching guidelines for these organizations and for comparison with the other organizations as highlighted.

Changing Paradigms

Caution is needed when reviewing older literature and understanding how shifts in diagnostic classification and the significance of molecular alterations (ie, RAS mutations) impact testing performance and treatment recommendations.[28,33] Trends toward more conservative approaches to thyroid cancer management over time have also impacted algorithms.[10] The recent reclassification of noninvasive follicular variant of papillary thyroid carcinoma to noninvasive follicular thyroid neoplasm with papillary like nuclei (NIFTP) is one such shift.[41,42] A subgroup of previously classified noninvasive encapsulated follicular variant of papillary thyroid carcinoma is no longer classified as malignant under this new nomenclature. However, as many NIFTP harbor mutations or fusions, this is still considered a neoplasm for which surgical lobectomy is considered both therapeutic and diagnostic. As biologic progression may theoretically occur, most testing algorithms choose to keep NIFTP in the true positive category as a likely premalignant lesion and shows better performance for detection.[6-8] More importantly, may be the increased recognition of molecular alterations in both benign and lower risk thyroid malignancies that would not independently warrant a total thyroidectomy. These shifting treatment algorithms allow for fewer total thyroidectomies based on assessed risk. More recent correlation with molecular alterations and those with distant metastases are beginning to inform future thyroid nodule risk stratification.

MOLECULAR VARIANCE BY CYTOLOGIC CLASSIFICATION

Understanding details of testing performance across platforms includes how the tests perform in Bethesda Category III versus Category IV and the inherent challenges and differences in testing when applied to FNAs with Hurthle features.[43,44]

Validation across platforms typically breaks down the results based on these 2 independent Bethesda cytology categories.[6,8,32] Slight performance differences can be attributed to lower rates of malignant disease in category III than category IV. Variations in pathologist classification of indeterminate nodules also may impact local performance.

MOLECULAR ASSESSMENT IN HURTHLE CELL RICH NODULES

Hurthle cell carcinoma, which represents ~5% of thyroid cancers, is molecularly complex with lower rates of common gene mutations and historically lower performance on per-operative molecular assessment by both approaches.[45,46] Early GEC found 86% of Hurthle cell nodules benign on surgical resection were "suspicious" by testing.[47-49] The GSC now shows enhanced performance with Hurthle nodules.[6] Moreover, modifications from thyroseq version 2 to version 3 were specifically added to augment the assay's performance in that unique subset by analyzing copy number and increasing the number of gene alterations assessed from 56 to 112 genes. Gene fusion coverage was also increased.[8] Although NCCN removed the caution note of poor performance in Hurthle cell nodules, continued data and application of these tests will likely be further refined.[13] This type of variation is a critical nuance that would be important to recognize when counseling patients, determining if and what type of testing may be warranted, and understanding that surgical triage for classification may still be warranted base on clinical and radiographic factors secondary to the degree of uncertainty that remains in Hurthle-based neoplasms.[50]

Commercial and Local Molecular Testing

The body of literature to validate testing performance accompanies commercially available testing for thyroid nodule assessment in the CLIA setting.[6-8] **Table 3** provides a broad view of testing performance in the most current versions of commercially available tests for thyroid-specific testing.[3-5] As highlighted, testing performance is still dependent on knowing the prevalence of malignancy in your local population.

Local molecular panels may be available in the CLIA setting for general oncologic tumor assessment; however, their performance in detecting thyroid malignancy may vary widely from the commercially thyroid-specific assays and the sensitivity and specificity will not be known without internal validation. More importantly will be to assess if the minimum 7-gene/fusion panel is included and assessing potential limitations of the local assay. such as if fusions are not included. The following critical factors should be considered before using and or counseling patients regarding local assays for thyroid nodule assessment for clinical triage. Are these assays permissible for FNA quantity size samples? What genomic alterations are included? Do they detect fusions and if so which ones? What is the threshold to report a mutation/alteration if present? How best to counsel a patient regarding assessment goals versus unknowns. Note that even with commercial molecular assays, that benefits, limitations, and unknowns exist (**Table 4**).

Multidisciplinary Approach

Timing for molecular collections requires multidisciplinary impute to optimize work-flow and unnecessary collections (FNA passes). Algorithms for when to perform an FNA collection for molecular testing need to consider that only indeterminate cytologic classification currently are typically tested, and be aware of patient factors that may warrant surgery regardless of testing. A workflow that includes immediate assessment by a cytopathologist may allow for triage to ancillary FNA sample collection for possible molecular testing in one setting when the initial cytologic assessment is falling into an indeterminate Bethesda category. Alternatively, collection as part of a follow-up visit may be beneficial allowing

Table 4
Molecular testing for indeterminate thyroid nodules

Benefits	• May be able to avoid surgery when a "rule-out" test with high negative predictive value (NPV) is negative • Newer testing platforms now have higher sensitivity for disease detection
Limitations	• The absence of molecular alterations in "rule-in" tests cannot entirely exclude malignancy • Molecular testing results would not negate other indications for surgical resection
Unknown	• Long-term follow-up to further validate testing performance for patients who did not proceed to surgery is needed

for the discussion of molecular testing with the patient in context of the Bethesda Category and cytologic findings (ie, Hurthle features). Note that ancillary collection for possible molecular testing may be held until after the final cytologic report confirms an indeterminate nodule and the input from the other clinical providers confirms the adjuvant role molecular testing may play for a patient's care. Commercial tests have collection kits and details regarding storage and shipping requirements on their websites.[3–5] Most methodologies require dedicated passes for molecular testing collection. Alternative testing materials beyond dedicated FNA passes into preservatives are being incorporated into some testing platforms (ie, testing from cell blocks, cytology slides) **Table 3**.

CONTINUED DISCUSSIONS

Discussions of the value of molecular testing in Category V suspicious nodules and even Category VI malignant nodules presurgery is debated. The identification of high-risk or a combination of mutations including p53 and/or TERT promoter mutations could augment algorithms for extent of the initial surgery for the small group of patients in whom this is identified.[23] Surgical alterations based on specific molecular alterations must ensure the risk benefit ratio is balanced. Further prospective studies and long-term follow-up will likely add to the literature enabling more informed decisions and refined algorithms in these settings.

SUMMARY

Although cytologic evaluation of thyroid nodules remains robust in 70% to 80% of cases, the 15% to 30% of cytologically indeterminate thyroid nodules (Bethesda Categories III and IV) remain clinically challenging.[15] Indeterminate categories show a wide range of malignant risk and historically only a surgical lobectomy could provide diagnostic confirmation of benign or malignant. Ancillary molecular testing designed specifically with thyroid nodules in mind may be used when the cytologic evaluation results in an indeterminate Bethesda category (III or IV). Although guidance varies across organizations (see **Box 1**), the common themes include that a negative molecular assessment should not alter the clinical determination if other factors advocate for surgical resection; when molecular alterations are detected there is a high likelihood of neoplasm; however, not all alterations screened for are synonymous with malignancy; and testing used should be performed in a CLIA laboratory and have a similar performance to reference benign cytology (ie, <5% risk of malignancy [rule-out type testing]). The decision for collection and sending molecular testing potential utility and benefit should be determined in conjunction with the treating team, allowing incorporation of other patient risk factors that may advocate for surgical removal regardless of molecular testing findings.

CLINICS CARE POINTS

- Prior to collecting/sending an FNA sample for molecular testing on an indeterminate thyroid nodule know the clinical scenario, testing methods' performance and assure council of the patient.

DISCLOSURE

The author has participated in scientific advisory boards for Bayer Pharmaceuticals (unrelated to this work).

REFERENCES

1. Bongiovanni M, Spitale A, Faquin WC, et al. The Bethesda System for reporting thyroid cytopathology: a meta-analysis. Acta Cytol 2012;56(4):333–9.
2. Melillo RM, Santoro M. Molecular biomarkers in thyroid FNA samples. J Clin Endocrinol Metab 2012; 97(12):4370–3.
3. Available at: https://www.afirma.com/physicians/. Accessed March 19, 2020.
4. Available at: https://thygenext-thyramir.com/. Accessed March 19, 2020.
5. Available at: https://thyroseq.com/home. Accessed March 19, 2020.
6. Patel KN, Angell TE, Babiarz J, et al. Performance of a genomic sequencing classifier for the preoperative diagnosis of cytologically indeterminate thyroid nodules. JAMA Surg 2018;153(9):817–24.
7. Lupo MA, Walts AE, Sistrunk JW, et al. Multiplatform molecular test performance in indeterminate thyroid nodules. Diagn Cytopathol 2020;48(12):1254–64.
8. Nikiforova MN, Mercurio S, Wald AI, et al. Analytical performance of the ThyroSeq v3 genomic classifier for cancer diagnosis in thyroid nodules. Cancer 2018;124:1682–90.
9. Krane JF, Cibas ES, Alexander EK, et al. Molecular analysis of residual ThinPrep material from thyroid FNAs increases diagnostic sensitivity. Cancer Cytopathol 2015;123:356–61.
10. Haugen BR, Alexander EK, Bible KC, et al. 2015 American Thyroid Association Management Guidelines for Adult Patients with Thyroid Nodules and Differentiated Thyroid Cancer: The American Thyroid Association Guidelines Task Force on Thyroid Nodules and Differentiated Thyroid Cancer. Thyroid 2016;26(1):1–133.
11. Francis GL, Waguespack SG, Bauer AJ, et al. Management guidelines for children with thyroid nodules and differentiated thyroid cancer American Thyroid Association guidelines task force. Thyroid 2015; 25(7):716–59.
12. Paschke R, Cantara S, Crescenzi A, et al. European Thyroid Association guidelines regarding thyroid nodule molecular fine-needle aspiration cytology diagnostics. Eur Thyroid J 2017;6(3):115–29.
13. Haddad RI, Bischoff L, Bernet V, et al. National Comprehensive Cancer Network. Clinical Practice Guidelines in Oncology. Thyroid carcinoma. Version 2.2020 – 2020. NCCN.org.
14. Gharib H, Papini E, Garber JR, et al. AACE/ACE/AME task force on thyroid nodules. American Association of Clinical Endocrinologists, American College of Endocrinology, and Associazione Medici Endocrinologi Medical guidelines for clinical practice for the diagnosis and management of thyroid nodules–2016 update. Endocr Pract 2016;22(5):622–39.
15. Baloch ZW, Cibas ES, Clark DP, et al. The National Cancer Institute thyroid fine needle aspiration state of the science conference: a summation. Cytojournal 2008;5:6.
16. Cibas ES, Ali SZ. The 2017 Bethesda system for reporting thyroid cytopathology. Thyroid 2017;27:1341–6.
17. Eilers SG, La Police P, Mukunyadzi P, et al. Thyroid fine-needle aspiration cytology: performance data of neoplastic and malignant cases as identified from 1558 responses in the ASCP Non-GYN assessment program thyroid fine-needle performance data. Cancer Cytopathol 2014;122:745–50.
18. Baloch ZW, Fleisher S, LiVolsi VA, et al. Diagnosis of "follicular neoplasm": a gray zone in thyroid fine-needle aspiration cytology. Diagn Cytopathol 2002;26:41–4.
19. Sherman SI. Thyroid carcinoma. Lancet 2003;361: 501–11.
20. Alexander EK, Kennedy GC, Baloch ZW, et al. Preoperative diagnosis of benign thyroid nodules with indeterminate cytology. N Engl J Med 2012;367(8):705–15.
21. Lastra RR, Pramick MR, Crammer CJ, et al. Implications of a suspicious afirma test result in thyroid fine-needle aspiration cytology: an institutional experience. Cancer Cytopathol 2014;122:737–44.
22. Marti JL, Avadhani V, Donatelli LA, et al. Wide inter-institutional variation in performance of a molecular classifier for indeterminate thyroid nodules. Ann Surg Oncol 2015;22:3996.
23. Cancer Genome Atlas Research Network. Integrated genomic characterization of papillary thyroid carcinoma. Cell 2014;159(3):676–90.
24. Sobrinho-Simões M, Máximo V, Rocha AS, et al. Intragenic mutations in thyroid cancer. Endocrinol Metab Clin North Am 2008;37:333–62.

25. Xing M. Molecular pathogenesis and mechanisms of thyroid cancer. Nat Rev Cancer 2013;13:184–99.

26. Trimboli P, Treglia G, Condorelli E, et al. BRAF-mutated carcinomas among thyroid nodules with prior indeterminate FNA report: a systematic review and meta-analysis. Clin Endocrinol (Oxf) 2016;84(3):315–20.

27. Yakushina VD, Lerner LV, Lavrov AV. Gene fusions in thyroid cancer. Thyroid 2018;28(2):158–67.

28. Nikiforov YE, Ohori NP, Hodak SP, et al. Impact of mutational testing on the diagnosis and management of patients with cytologically indeterminate thyroid nodules: a prospective analysis of 1056 FNA samples. J Clin Endocrinol Metab 2011;96:3390–7.

29. Bardet S, Goardon N, Lequesne J, et al. Diagnostic and prognostic value of a 7-panel mutation testing in thyroid nodules with indeterminate cytology: the SWEETMAC study. Endocrine 2021;71(2):407–17.

30. Nikiforova MN, Wald AI, Roy S, et al. Targeted next-generation sequencing panel (ThyroSeq) for detection of mutations in thyroid cancer. J Clin Endocrinol Metab 2013;98(11):E1852–60.

31. Nikiforov YE, Carty SE, Chiosea SI, et al. Highly accurate diagnosis of cancer in thyroid nodules with follicular neoplasm/suspicious for a follicular neoplasm cytology by ThyroSeq v2 next-generation sequencing assay. Cancer 2014;120(23):3627–34.

32. Nikiforov YE, Carty SE, Chiosea SI, et al. Impact of the multi-gene ThyroSeq Next-generation sequencing assay on cancer diagnosis in thyroid nodules with atypia of undetermined significance/follicular lesion of undetermined significance cytology. Thyroid 2015;25(11):1217–23.

33. Goldner WS, Angell TE, McAdoo SL, et al. Molecular variants and their risks for malignancy in cytologically indeterminate thyroid nodules. Thyroid 2019;29(11):1594–605.

34. Valderrabano P, Khazai L, Thompson ZJ, et al. Impact of oncogene panel results on surgical management of cytologically indeterminate thyroid nodules. Head Neck 2018;40(8):1812–23.

35. Ravella L, Lopez J, Descotes F, et al. Preoperative role of RAS or BRAF K601E in the guidance of surgery for indeterminate thyroid nodules. World J Surg 2020;44(7):2264–71.

36. Jackson S, Kumar G, Banizs AB, et al. Incremental utility of expanded mutation panel when used in combination with microRNA classification in indeterminate thyroid nodules. Diagn Cytopathol 2020;48(1):43–52.

37. Labourier E, Shifrin A, Busseniers AE, et al. Molecular testing for miRNA, mRNA, and DNA on fine-needle aspiration improves the preoperative diagnosis of thyroid nodules with indeterminate cytology. J Clin Endocrinol Metab 2015;100(7):2743–50.

38. Monaco SE, Pantanowitz L, Khalbuss WE, et al. Cytomorphological and molecular genetic findings in pediatric thyroid fine-needle aspiration. Cancer Cytopathol 2012;120:342–50.

39. Buryk MA, Monaco SE, Witchel SF, et al. Preoperative cytology with molecular analysis to help guide surgery for pediatric thyroid nodules. Int J Pediatr Otorhinolaryngol 2013;77:1697–700.

40. Picarsic JL, Buryk MA, Ozolek J, et al. Molecular characterization of sporadic pediatric thyroid carcinoma with the DNA/RNA ThyroSeq v2 next-generation sequencing assay. Pediatr Dev Pathol 2016;19(2):115–22.

41. Baloch ZW, Seethala RR, Faquin WC, et al. Noninvasive follicular thyroid neoplasm with papillary-like nuclear features (NIFTP): a changing paradigm in thyroid surgical pathology and implications for thyroid cytopathology. Cancer Cytopathol 2016;124:616–20.

42. Faquin WC, Wong LQ, Afrogheh AH, et al. Impact of reclassifying noninvasive follicular variant of papillary thyroid carcinoma on the risk of malignancy in the Bethesda System for Reporting Thyroid Cytopathology. Cancer Cytopathol 2016;124:181–7.

43. Steward DL, Carty SE, Sippel RS, et al. Performance of a multigene genomic classifier in thyroid nodules with indeterminate cytology A prospective blinded multicenter study. JAMA Oncol 2019;5(2):204–12.

44. Nikiforov YE, Baloch ZW. Clinical validation of the ThyroSeq v3 genomic classifier in thyroid nodules with indeterminate FNA cytology. Cancer Cytopathol 2019;127(4):225–30.

45. Ganly I, Makarov V, Deraje S, et al. Integrated genomic analysis of Hurthle cell cancer reveals oncogenic drivers, recurrent mitochondrial mutations, and unique chromosomal landscapes. Cancer Cell 2018;34(2):256–70.

46. Gopal RK, Kübler K, Calvo SE, et al. Widespread chromosomal losses and mitochondrial DNA alterations as genetic drivers in Hurthle cell carcinoma. Cancer Cell 2018;34(2):242–55.

47. McIver B, Castro MR, Morris JC, et al. An independent study of a gene expression classifier (Afirma) in the evaluation of cytologically indeterminate thyroid nodules. J Clin Endocrinol Metab 2014;99:4069–77.

48. Celik B, Whetsell CR, Nassar A. Afirma GEC and thyroid lesions: an institutional experience. Diagn Cytopathol 2015;43:966–70.

49. Brauner E, Holmes BJ, Krane JF, et al. Performance of the Afirma gene expression classifier in Hurthle cell thyroid nodules differs from other indeterminate thyroid nodules. Thyroid 2015;25:789–96.

50. Jalaly JB, Baloch ZW. Hürthle-cell neoplasms of the thyroid: an algorithmic approach to pathologic diagnosis in light of molecular advances. Semin Diagn Pathol 2020;37(5):234–42.

51. Krane JF, Cibas ES, Endo M, et al. The Afirma Xpression Atlas for thyroid nodules and thyroid cancer metastases: insights to inform clinical decision-making from a fine-needle aspiration sample. Cancer Cytopathol 2020;128(7):452–9.

Imaging of Cervical Lymph Nodes in Thyroid Cancer
Ultrasound and Computed Tomography

Noah Nathan Chasen, MD[a], Jennifer Rui Wang, MD, ScM[b], Qiong Gan, MD[c],
Salmaan Ahmed, MD[a,*]

KEYWORDS

• PTC • Ultrasound • FNA • Metastatic adenopathy • Metastatic mimics • Preoperative staging

KEY POINTS

• Preoperative imaging in all patients with thyroid cancer should include a detailed sonographic evaluation of central compartment (CC) (levels VI and VII) and lateral compartment (LC) (levels I–IV and V) lymph nodes.
• CC metastases are resected via the thyroidectomy incision, whereas LC metastasis requires the addition of lateral neck dissection. Therefore, the presence of lateral neck metastasis should be confirmed via preoperative fine-needle aspiration (FNA) biopsy.
• Thyroglobulin test of the FNA sample can increase sensitivity and should be obtained with cystic lymph nodes and when lymph nodes with suspicious imaging features yield benign or nondiagnostic cytology.
• Contrast-enhanced computed tomography of the neck is complementary to gray-scale ultrasound with Doppler in the staging of thyroid cancer. Postoperative administration of radioiodine can be delayed 6 weeks to 8 weeks to allow for clearance of iodine load from computed tomography contrast.
• Presence of high-level VI nodal metastases above the thyroid gland and medial to the carotid artery should be communicated specifically to the surgeon, because CC resection is not extended routinely cranial to the inferior thyroid artery.

INTRODUCTION

Papillary, medullary, poorly differentiated, and anaplastic thyroid carcinomas commonly metastasize to cervical lymph nodes, whereas nodal metastases are uncommon in follicular thyroid carcinoma.[1,2] Preoperative evaluation of cervical lymph nodes may alter the surgical procedure in a significant proportion of patients. As such, all patients diagnosed with thyroid cancer should undergo, at minimum, preoperative ultrasound (US) evaluation of bilateral central and lateral neck lymph nodes. Several recent studies have shown a complementary role of contrast-enhanced computed tomography (CECT) when combined with US in patients with cervical lymph node metastasis from papillary thyroid carcinoma (PTC).[3] Therefore, patients with clinically palpable, suspicious nodes on US and/or cytologically confirmed lateral neck nodal disease require further evaluation using CECT neck to determine extent of disease and surgical resectability.[4]

[a] Department of Neuroradiology, The University of Texas MD Anderson Cancer Center, 1515 Holcombe Boulevard, Unit 1482, Houston, TX 77030-4009, USA; [b] Department of Head and Neck Surgery, The University of Texas MD Anderson Cancer Center, 1515 Holcombe Boulevard, Unit 1445, Houston, TX 77030-4009, USA; [c] Department of Anatomical Pathology, The University of Texas MD Anderson Cancer Center, 1515 Holcombe Boulevard, Unit 0085, Houston, TX 77030-4009, USA
* Corresponding author.
E-mail address: salmaan.ahmed@mdanderson.org

Neuroimag Clin N Am 31 (2021) 313–326
https://doi.org/10.1016/j.nic.2021.04.002
1052-5149/21/© 2021 Elsevier Inc. All rights reserved.

CECT neck also provides evaluation of retropharyngeal lymph nodes (LRNs), which may be involved in patients with PTC.[5] Moreover, additional imaging, including CECT neck, should be obtained in patients with locally advanced disease (ie, vocal cord paralysis, extrathyroidal extension, or substernal extension) and/or concerns for aggressive histology, such as poorly differentiated or anaplastic thyroid carcinoma. Postoperative administration of radioactive iodine can be delayed 6 weeks to 8 weeks because contrast administration alters radioactive iodine uptake for 6 weeks to 8 weeks. Because it is similar in accuracy to computed tomography (CT) in the evaluation of locally aggressive disease, magnetic resonance imaging (MRI) of the neck is useful in patients where iodinated contrast is contraindicated, such as in severe allergy, in renal dysfunction, or when radioactive iodine ablation cannot be delayed.[2] Otherwise, in the absence of any contraindication to intravenous iodine and with the availability of CT and US, there is less utility for MRI in the preoperative nodal evaluation in patients with thyroid malignancy.[6,7]

ANATOMY

The current imaging classification system provides reproducible landmarks of the regional lymph nodes that are compatible with the clinical staging used by the American Academy of Otolaryngology–Head and Neck Surgery and the American Joint Committee on Cancer (AJCC).[8] The cervical lymph nodes are grouped into 7 regions or levels (Fig. 1). Level I includes the clinically classified submental (IA) and submandibular (IB) lymph nodes, which are separated by the anterior belly of the digastric muscle. Both levels IA and IB are bordered superiorly by the mylohyoid muscle, inferiorly by the hyoid bone, and posteriorly by the posterior border of the submandibular gland. Levels II, III, and IV nodes are clinically termed the upper, middle, and lower jugular nodes, respectively. On imaging, level II is bordered superiorly by the skull base, inferiorly by the hyoid bone, anteriorly by the back of the submandibular gland, and posteriorly by the posterior border of the sternocleidomastoid muscle (SCM). Level III nodes are bordered superiorly by the hyoid and inferiorly by the lower cricoid arch. Level IV nodes are located superior to the clavicle, inferior to the lower cricoid, and lateral to the medial wall of the CCA. Level V nodes are separated into levels Va and Vb by the lower cricoid cartilage. Level Va comprises nodes from the skull base to the level of the lower cricoid and are located posterior to the posterior border of the SCM. Level Vb nodes are located inferior to the

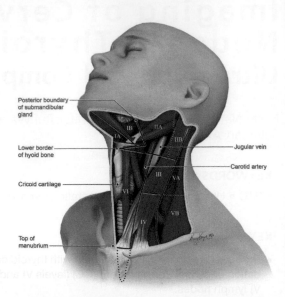

Fig. 1. Nodal compartments in the neck. (*Courtesy of* K, Kage, BS, MFA, Houston, Texas.)

cricoid, superior to the clavicle, and posterolateral to the plane connecting the anterolateral wall of the anterior scalene to the posterior SCM border. Level VI is clinically classified as nodes within the CC or visceral space and includes those at greatest risk for metastasis from thyroid cancer. This group is bounded superiorly by the lower hyoid, inferiorly by the suprasternal notch and laterally by the medial sheaths of the carotid arteries. Level VI includes paratracheal, pretracheal, perithyroidal, and precricoid (Delphian) nodes. Level VII nodes are in the superior mediastinum below the suprasternal notch. They are bounded inferiorly by the innominate vein.[9]

TECHNIQUE

US scanning of the soft tissues of the neck should be performed with a high-resolution US scanner (Sequoia, Acuson, Mountain View, California; Elegra, Siemens, Issaquah, Washington; HDI 5000, Philips–ATL, Bothell, Washington; or PowerVision 7000, Toshiba, Tokyo, Japan) equipped with a high-frequency linear-array transducer of at least 7 MHz and up to 13 MHz. Examination protocol includes a detailed evaluation of the thyroid as well a comprehensive evaluation of the cervical lymph nodes including the central compartment (CC) (levels VI and VII), lateral compartment (LC) (levels II, III, IV, and V), and also the submental and submandibular region (level I).[10] CECT neck for the evaluation of thyroid malignancy is complementary to US and can be performed on a 4-detector to 16-detector LightSpeed CT scanner (GE Healthcare, Milwaukee, Wisconsin), with axial 1.25-mm

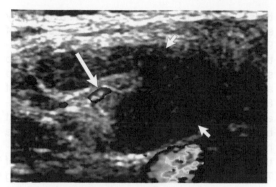

Fig. 2. GSCUD of a normal lymph node shows a central echogenic hilum with hilar vascularity (*long arrow*). The hypoechoic cortex (*short arrows*) is similar in echogenicity to strap muscle.

to 3-mm collimation at 120 kVp and 160 mA to 400 mA, after injection of 125 mL of Omnipaque 350 (GE Healthcare) at 3 mL/s with a 90-second delay.[11]

NORMAL LYMPH NODES

A normal lymph node is a kidney-bean shaped organ of the lymphatic system, which has a convex surface that is penetrated by afferent lymph vessels. On the opposing side, the concave hilum is penetrated by the supplying artery, vein, and nerve as well as the efferent lymphatic vessels with variable amount of fatty tissue. Histologically, lymph nodes are encapsulated by dense capsule, and the cross-section of a lymph node consists of 3 major areas or zones: the cortex, paracortex, and medulla (**Fig. 2**). The cortex is located peripherally, below the capsule, and consists of lymphoid follicles of different sizes. The medulla, the deepest

layer of lymph node, is rich in arteries, veins and a minor lymphocytic component. The paracortex, between the cortex and medulla, contains a mobile pool of T-lymphocytes.

Sonographically, normal lymph nodes (see **Fig. 2**) are oval, with a peripheral cortex hypoechoic to the strap muscles, with a central echogenic hilum, and with central hilar vascularity.[12] Normal lymph nodes lack calcifications, cystic change, and necrosis.[13] Although rounded configuration and overall enlargement of nodes are indicators of malignancy, the size and shape of normal cervical nodes vary with location. Submandibular and level II lymph nodes tend to be larger than the lymph nodes in the lower neck. Normal submandibular and parotid lymph nodes often demonstrate a rounded configuration.[12]

MALIGNANT LYMPH NODES

Cervical metastatic lymph nodes demonstrate pathologic alterations, which may be detected sonographically and with CT. Small foci of tumor deposit within the cortex or near the hilum could be seen as cortical thickening with altered echogenicity (**Fig. 3**). Growth of tumor within the lymph node results in enlargement especially along the short axis leading to a rounded shape, hilar obliteration (**Fig. 4**), and increased vascularity.[14]

Psammomatous calcifications thought to be due to infarcted tips of malignant papillae seen under microscope manifest as punctate hyperechogenic foci on US (**Fig. 5**). Cystic change (**Fig. 6**) in metastatic lymph nodes, resulting from degeneration of tumor cells or from colloid secretion, is associated with metastatic adenopathy of PTC.[15] Intranodal calcification (see **Fig. 5**; **Fig. 7**) and cystic change (see **Fig. 6**) have been shown to

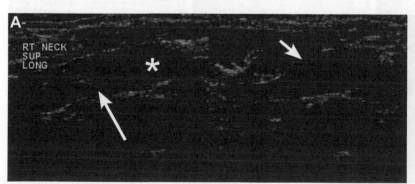
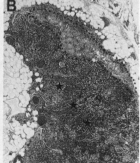

Fig. 3. (*A*) Longitudinal (*left image*) and transverse (*right image*) GSU image in a 43-year-old man shows a right level II node with focal, asymmetric hypoechoic expansion of the cortex (*star*) and preservation of the normal echogenic hilum (*arrow*) and normal echotexture to the remaining cortex. FNA, metastatic PTC. (*B*) Pathology hematoxylin-eosin stain (original magnification ×20) of a representative lymph node from a different patient with focal cortical metastatic PTC (*dotted border*) within an otherwise preserved normal node (*stars*).

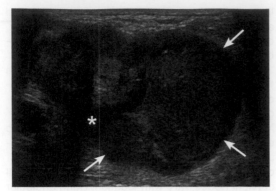

Fig. 4. GSU of a 4-cm left level IV metastasis in a 70-year-old woman with PTC shows nodal enlargement with diffuse abnormal hypoechogenicity to the cortex (*arrows*), loss of the normal hilum, and a small cystic component (*asterisk*).

have specificity greater than 90%[16–18] with some studies demonstrating 100% specificity for metastatic differentiated thyroid carcinoma.[14,17] Because the sensitivity of punctate hyperechoic calcification and cystic changes usually is less than 50%,[14,16,17,19] however, the absence of these features should not deter lymph node sampling in the presence of other worrisome findings.

Metastatic nodal echogenicity can be described generally as abnormal[19] versus hyperechoic (Fig. 8) [8,14,17,20,21] or hypoechoic (see Fig. 4)[13] compared with muscle. The sensitivity for nodal hyperechogenicity as a malignant feature in patients with PTC ranges from 55% to 86% and specificity from 70% to 95.5%.[14,17,21] For example, a review of 350 lymph nodes in 112 patients with PTC using hyperechogenicity relative

to strap muscle as a marker for malignancy showed a sensitivity of 86% and a specificity of 95.5%.[17] A review of 1976 lymph nodes in 118 patients evaluating hypoechogenicity relative to strap muscle as a marker for malignancy showed a sensitivity of 90.9% and a specificity of 83.3%.[13] The relative lower specificity using hypoechogenicity likely is explained by the fact that both normal and reactive lymph nodes can be hypoechoic, whereas hyperechoic normal or reactive nodes are uncommon.[17] Another review of 767 lymph nodes (109 patients with PTC) using abnormal echogenicity as a marker for malignancy, without further specifying if hyperechoic or hypoechoic, demonstrated a sensitivity of 82.4 and specificity of 77.2 for detecting nodal metastasis.[19] Therefore, when staging patients with PTC, lymph nodes with general abnormal echotexture can be selected for fine-needle aspiration (FNA).

Absence of an echogenic hilum (see Figs. 5, 7, and 8) is highly sensitive for malignancy, with sensitivity that ranged from 88% to 93% and specificity that ranged from 53% to 90%.[13,17,19] The lower specificity may be explained by the fact that certain normal and inflammatory nodes may not display a hilum.[16,22]

Lymph nodes with an index value (short axis/long axis) greater than 0.5 have 71% to 89% specificity for metastasis,[14,17,19,23] although there is a wide range in the sensitivity from 24% to 80%. Therefore, although lymph nodes with a rounded configuration can be regarded as suspicious (see Fig. 5; Fig. 9), the presence of an oval configuration should not deter FNA when other concerning features are present.

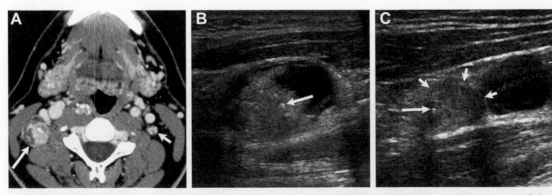

Fig. 5. (*A*) CECT in a 30-year-old man demonstrates a 2.3-cm right level IIA node (*large arrow*) and a 1-cm left level IIB lymph node (*small arrow*), both with enhancement, cystic changes, and calcifications. Right LRN metastasis is noted. (*B*) On GSU, the right level IIA lymph node is predominantly solid, hyperechoic to muscle with a cystic component, and contains punctate calcification (*arrow*). (*C*) GSU of the left level IIB node (*short arrows*) demonstrates solid hyperechoic echotexture with microcalcification (*long arrow*). Surgical pathology from bilateral neck dissection = metastatic PTC.

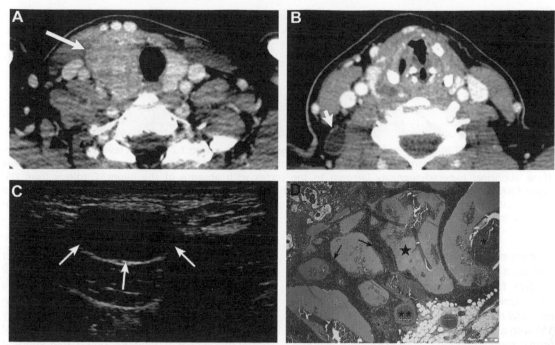

Fig. 6. (*A*) Axial CECT image in a 39-year-old demonstrates a solid 5-cm heterogeneous right thyroid mass (*long arrow*). (*B*) CECT image in the same patient as in figure A shows a right level IV cystic node (*small arrow*). (*C*) GSUD of the right level IV node shows an anechoic cystic lesion (*long arrows*) without soft tissue nodularity (or not shown). FNA right lobe mass = PTC. FNA of the right level IV node yielded 10 mL of cloudy/bloody fluid with cytology = metastatic PTC. (*D*) Hematoxylin-eosin (original magnification ×40) histology from cystic PTC nodal metastasis in a different patient demonstrates areas of cystic contents containing colloid (*star*) surrounded by a thin layer of PTC follicular cells (*arrows*) that are surrounded by several layers of lymphocytes. Internal cystic hemorrhage (*) and a dilated vessel (**) are noted.

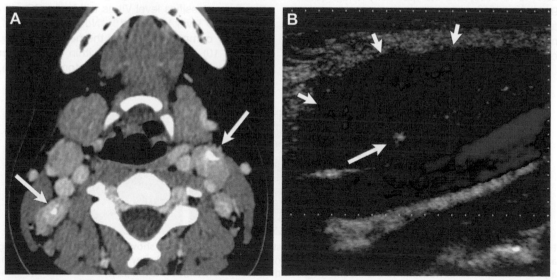

Fig. 7. (*A*) Axial CECT in a 15-year-old girl with PTC shows bilateral level II nodal metastasis (*arrows*) with coarse calcifications. (*B*) Concurrent GSUD of the right level II lymph node demonstrates abnormal hypoechogenicity, expansion of the cortex (*short arrows*), and disorganized vascular flow. Central hyperechogenic foci correspond to coarse calcifications (*long arrow*) and should not be confused with an echogenic hilum, which is absent in this case.

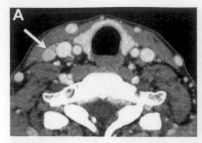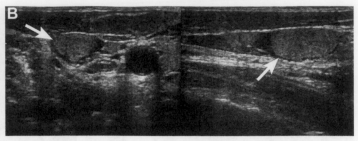

Fig. 8. (A) Axial CECT in 43-year-old woman with PTC shows an enhancing 1.2-cm right level IV lymph node (arrow). (B) Concurrent transverse (left image) GSU and longitudinal (right image) images of the node (A) shows diffuse abnormal hyperechogenicity (arrows) to the cortex with absence of the hilum. Cytology from US-guided FNA shows atypical thyroid follicular cells with nuclear enlargement and few nuclear grooves and a rare intranuclear inclusion surrounded by small and large fragments of inspissated colloid, suspicious for metastatic PTC (not shown).

Lymph node long axis greater than or equal to 1 cm as a marker for malignancy was only 68% sensitive for PTC metastasis with 75% specificity.[16] Using short axis greater than 5 mm to predict nodal metastasis demonstrated a sensitivity of 61% with a specificity of 96%.[16] Therefore, no size cutoff is recommended to screen for cervical nodal metastasis from PTC, and selection for FNA should be based on morphology.

A retrospective study evaluating abnormal nodal vascularity (nonhilar and mixed vascularity) as a marker for metastatic PTC (see Figs. 7B and 9C) demonstrated greater than 95% specificity, although sensitivity was only 53%.[24] When peripheral vascularity is used as an isolated criteria for nodal malignancy, the sensitivity is relatively low, at 47% to 76%, and the specificity is high (57%–99%),[13,14,19,23]; therefore, the presence of abnormal vascularity is highly suspicious for nodal metastasis whereas the absence is not reliable for exclusion.

Although grey scale ultrasound with Doppler (GSUD) is the modality of choice for the initial evaluation in thyroid malignancy, CECT of the neck plays a complementary role.[2,25] The presence of central necrosis on CECT is nearly 100% accurate in predicting the presence of nodal metastasis.[26] Findings on CT that suggest nodal metastasis secondary to PTC include cystic changes, calcification, and avid enhancement.[2,27]

PREOPERATIVE STAGING/PATTERNS OF CERVICAL NODAL METASTASIS

The CC (levels VI/VII) is considered the first echelon of nodal metastases in thyroid cancer.[25] The updated AJCC Cancer Staging Manual, eighth edition, now classifies level VII as within the CC,[28] in addition to level VI (Fig. 10). Nodal levels II, III, IV, and V comprise the LC of the neck (see Figs. 9C and 10). Neck dissection within the CC can be performed via the thyroidectomy incision,

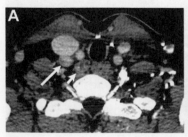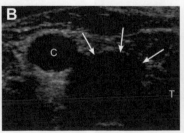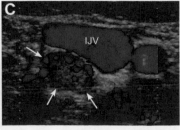

Fig. 9. (A) Axial CECT in a 46-year-old woman status post-thyroidectomy for PTC shows 2 metastatic nodes (long arrow and short arrow) in the right inferior neck, posterior to carotid sheath. (B) grey scale ultrasound (GSU) image of the right lower neck shows the medial lymph node (short arrow [A]) is located posteromedial to the common carotid artery (C), and will require central neck dissection. US allows for precise localization of the node (arrows) as level VI, between the carotid artery (C) and the trachea (T). (C) GSUD of the lateral node (long arrow [A]) confirms this node (arrows) as level IV: posterolateral to the carotid and IJV. Resection of this node is achieved via lateral neck dissection requiring a separate incision from that required for central neck dissection. Surgical pathology = metastatic PTC.

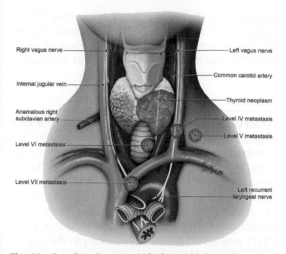

Fig. 10. Graphic showing left thyroid lobe malignancy with left CC (levels VI and VII) nodal metastasis located medial to the common carotid artery and left LC (levels IV and V) nodal metastasis located lateral to the common carotid artery. There is an aberrant right subclavian artery, which is associated with a right nonrecurrent laryngeal nerve. (*Courtesy of* K, Kage, BS, MFA, Houston, Texas.)

whereas removal of nodes in the LC is achieved via extension to a lateral neck dissection. The landmark that separates the central and lateral compartments is the medial margin of the common carotid artery, which is identified 'more easily on axial images than the traditional intraoperative lateral border of the sternohyoid muscle.[29] In the LC, metastases commonly involve levels II to V.[30] Suspicious appearing lymph nodes identified on US and/or CT should be subjected to US-guided FNA, particularly in the LC, to facilitate complete resection of tumor burden at the initial surgery.

Although core needle biopsy does not appear to provide additional diagnostic benefit compared with FNA in PTC, it may be beneficial for the diagnosis of poorly differentiated and anaplastic thyroid carcinomas, particularly when molecular testing is required.[11,31] Core biopsy also may be used to rule out other diagnoses, such as lymphoma.

Thyroglobulin (Tg) measurement on lymph node FNA specimens has been shown to improve the sensitivity of FNA cytology in PTC (see Fig. 12), even in the presence of circulating anti-Tg antibodies.[32] This is useful particularly in cases of cystic nodal disease, where FNA cytology is nondiagnostic and only demonstrates foamy macrophages (Figs. 11B, C; see Fig. 12A, B). Lymph nodes with micrometastasis may demonstrate benign cytology, and Tg testing of the aspirate can be obtained when imaging features on CT or US are discordant with FNA cytology. Metastatic nodes with dense calcification may yield nondiagnostic cytology, and Tg testing of the aspirate can increase sensitivity (see Fig. 12C, D).

SPECIAL CONSIDERATIONS
Transoral Biopsy of Retropharyngeal Lymph Nodes

CECT is useful in detecting LRN metastasis from PTC, which is not evaluated on US. Transoral biopsy of LRN (see Fig. 11C) may be considered if pathologic confirmation of metastatic disease is needed for surgical planning.[33]

Aberrant Anatomy

The nonrecurrent laryngeal nerve is a rare (<1%) anatomic variation of the recurrent laryngeal nerve where the nerve enters the larynx off of the vagus

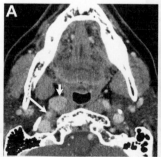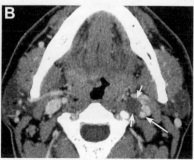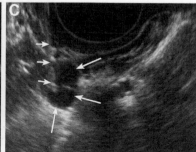

Fig. 11. (*A*) Axial CECT in a 71-year-old man with newly diagnosed PTC shows a 1.8-cm enhancing rounded right LRN (*short arrow*) medial to the internal carotid artery (*long arrow*). (*B*) Axial CECT in a 47-year-old man with recurrent PTC 8 years after initial thyroidectomy and bilateral central and lateral neck dissections, shows a cystic left LRN metastasis (*short arrows*) anteromedial to the internal carotid artery (*long arrow*). (*C*) Transoral GSU image acquired during FNA of the left LRN. The biopsy needle is seen as a thin echogenic stripe (*short arrows*) traversing the soft tissues of the upper oropharynx into the anechoic cystic node (*long arrows*), which demonstrates posterior acoustic enhancement.

nerve without descending into the thorax.[34] This typically occurs on the right side. In most cases, the nonrecurrent laryngeal nerve is associated with an aberrant right subclavian artery (see **Fig. 10**). Presence of a nonrecurrent laryngeal nerve can be a risk factor for iatrogenic injury during surgical resection. Although a systematic and careful dissection enables identification of this anatomic variant by experienced thyroid surgeons, identification of an aberrant subclavian artery on preoperative CT can draw the surgeon's attention to the possibility of a nonrecurrent laryngeal nerve, which facilitates intraoperative identification.[35]

High-level VI Nodal Metastasis

Some investigators recommend that the superior border of the CC neck dissection be defined by the inferior thyroid artery and a plane at the level of the cricoid cartilage or by a line demarcating the entrance point of the recurrent laryngeal nerve into the cricothyroid membrane,[36,37] because metastatic lymph nodes rarely are found cephalad to

the artery and this approach minimizes risk of injury to the superior parathyroid glands. Failure to communicate the specific presence of high-level VI nodal metastasis can result in incomplete resection (**Fig. 13**).

Vascular Encasement/Invasion

Direct lateral extension of the primary tumor and/or coalescing LC lymphadenopathy can encase the common carotid or internal carotid artery with an impact on resectability.[38] Macroscopic tumor spread into the internal jugular vein (IJV) (**Fig. 14**) can occur from disease spreading along the draining veins of the thyroid or from vascular invasion by extracapsular spread of PTC nodal metastasis.[38,39] CECT and GSUD are complementary in the evaluation of vascular encasement and venous invasion.[38–40]

Intraoperative Ultrasound Localization

In treatment-naïve patients, comprehensive neck dissection is performed to address nodal disease

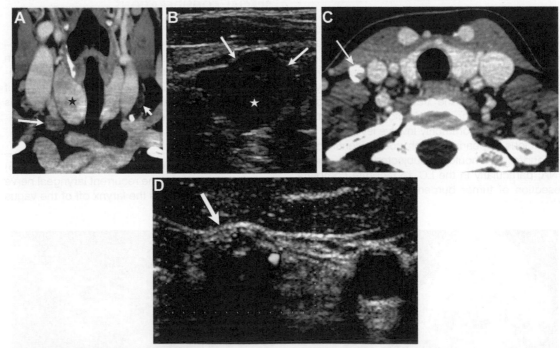

Fig. 12. (A) Coronal CECT in a 28-year-old woman with right lobe PTC (*star*) and right 1.6-cm right lateral compartment metastasis (*long arrow*). There is a 1.4-cm left level IV cystic node (*short arrow*). (B) Concurrent GSUD of the 1.4-cm left level IV node with abnormal cortex (*long arrows*) and cystic changes (*star*) was without malignant cells on preliminary cytology after FNA. Tg test performed on additional FNA sample returned 3984 ng/mL, confirming metastatic PTC. (C) Preoperative axial CECT in a 46-year-old woman with PTC shows a densely calcified 9-mm right level IV node (*arrow*), suspicious for metastasis. (D) Concurrent GSUD of the 9-mm calcified node (A) shows abnormal echotexture with multiple hyperechogenic foci (*arrow*) and with abnormal vascularity. Subsequent FNA = nondiagnostic preliminary cytology. Given the highly suspicious imaging features, Tg test of repeat FNA was obtained and returned Tg = 3431 ng/mL, compatible with metastasis. Right neck dissection demonstrated metastatic PTC on surgical pathology.

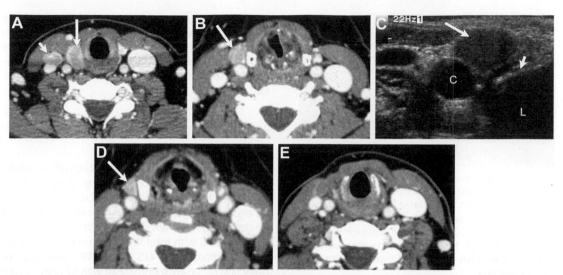

Fig. 13. (*A*) Preoperative axial CECT in a 51-year-old woman with FNA of 2-cm nodule in the right upper thyroid (*long arrow*) demonstrating PTC. Enhancing enlarged right level IV node was biopsied as metastatic PTC (*short arrow*). (*B*) Axial CECT in the same patient at a level superior to the thyroid shows a 1.5-cm enhancing node (*arrow*) anterior to the carotid artery, which may represent level III versus level VI metastasis. (*C*) Concurrent transverse GSU of the nodule (*B*) confirms a solid rounded hypoechoic node (*long arrow*) medial to the carotid artery (*C*) and lateral to the echogenic thyroid cartilage (*short arrow*) and larynx (L). This high-level VI node is not included routinely in a CC neck dissection, because it lies above the inferior thyroid artery which some surgeons use as the cranial resection margin. (*D, E*) Follow-up CECT in the same patient performed 1 year after thyroidectomy and right neck dissection shows residual high right level VI metastasis (*arrow*). FNA = metastatic PTC, which was subsequently resected. The presence of high-level VI metastasis should be communicated specifically to the surgeon because this region is not resected routinely during CC because of risk to the upper parathyroid gland blood supply and the relative low incidence of disease in this location. (*E*) There is no recurrence in the thyroidectomy beds or in the right lateral neck.

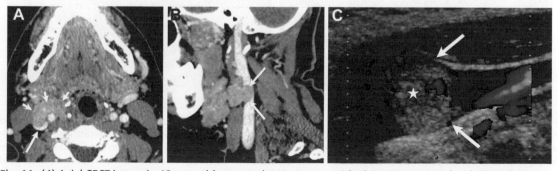

Fig. 14. (*A*) Axial CECT image in 46-year-old woman demonstrates residual 3-cm metastatic level II lymphadenopathy (*small arrows*) 2 months following thyroidectomy, resulting in partial effacement of the IJV (*long arrow*) secondary to external compression or direct invasion. (*B*) Sagittal CECT confirms effacement of the IJV (*arrows*), although it is difficult to differentiate IJV compression versus direct invasion. (*C*) Longitudinal GSUD shows echogenic solid tumor with internal vascularity (*star*) between both hyperechoic vessel walls (*arrows*) with luminal expansion, which confirms direct invasion of the IJV.

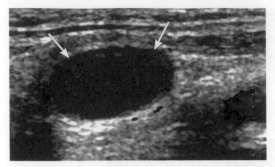

Fig. 15. A 25-year-old man with PTC status post-thyroidectomy, central neck dissection, and left lateral neck dissection; 11 years later, patient underwent right lateral neck dissection for recurrence. Postoperative follow-up GSUD shows an enlarging, hypoechoic, left midneck 1.3-cm node, with absence of the hilum (arrows). FNA = lymphoid tissue with no metastatic carcinoma.

in the neck. In recurrent disease, however, where prior comprehensive neck dissection has been performed, intraoperative US localization may be helpful to precisely localize the biopsy-proved disease, particularly if the disease is not large volume and difficult to locate.[41]

POSTOPERATIVE SURVEILLANCE OF THE NECK

Although PTC generally is associated with excellent prognosis, recurrence occurs in up to 30% of patients.[42] It has been shown that US performed by an experienced operator is the most sensitive tool for detecting recurrent disease in the neck.[43] In patients treated with total thyroidectomy and radioiodine ablation, neck US was 94% sensitive for detecting recurrence compared with 57% for serum Tg measurement and 45% for diagnostic ^{131}I whole-

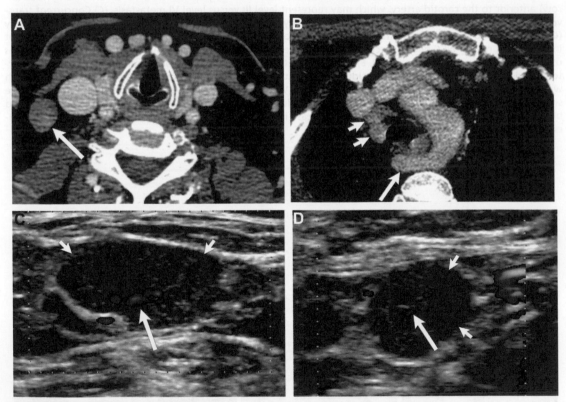

Fig. 16. (A) Axial CECT in a 57-year-old woman with PTC involving isthmus and rounded, homogenous, enlarged right level III node (arrow). (B) Axial CECT image at the superior mediastinum shows right paratracheal adenopathy (small arrows) and incidental aberrant right subclavian artery (long arrow). (C) Concurrent GSUD of the node in (A) shows an enlarged hypoechoic node (small arrows) with absence of the hilum and preserved central vascular flow (long arrow). (D) GSUD shows a rounded level II node (short arrows) with abnormal hypoechogenicity, absence of the hilum and preserved central vascular flow (long arrow). The nodes ([C] and [D]) both were biopsied without malignant cells and demonstrate lymphoid tissue with histiocyte collections and granulomatous change. Subsequent transbronchial biopsy of mediastinal nodes shows lymphoid tissue with non-necrotizing granulomas, raising concern for sarcoid. Patient was treated with thyroidectomy only and did not require neck dissection.

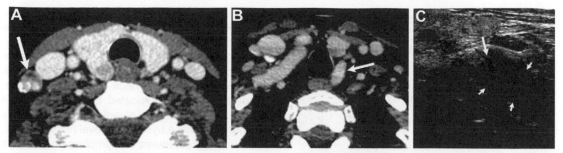

Fig. 17. (*A*) Axial CECT in a 63-year-old woman with right lobe PTC and right level IV nodal metastasis (*arrow*). (*B*) Axial CECT image in the same patient shows a 1.6-cm left paratracheal enhancing nodule, which may represent level VI nodal metastasis versus a parathyroid lesion (*arrow*). (*C*) GSUD of the left suprasternal neck shows a hypoechoic (*short arrows*) solid nodule (*long arrow* [*B*]) (*short arrows*) with a polar vessel (*long arrow*), favoring parathyroid lesion. Pathology = nodular parathyroid hyperplasia.

body scan, respectively.[44] Depending on risk stratification, surveillance neck US is performed at 6-month to 12-month intervals along with measurement of Tg levels. Although US findings can be highly suggestive of recurrence, US-guided FNA is necessary for pathologic confirmation.

If biochemical or US evidence of recurrence is identified, other imaging modalities are added to identify location of disease. CECT neck is most useful for assessment of recurrent neck disease, whereas MRI and PET/CT are used to identify distant metastases.

THYROID CANCER MIMICS

Reactive (**Fig. 15**), inflammatory, and granulomatous nodes may mimic metastasis from thyroid cancer. Reactive nodes usually are found in the high jugular (level II) or submandibular (level I) regions of the neck,[22,45] and sonographic features include oval shape, hypoechoic cortex, preservation of the echogenic hilum, and presence of central hilar vasculature.[8,22,45]

Lymphadenopathy secondary to sarcoidosis (**Fig. 16**) and tuberculosis can cause chronic granulomatous changes with intranodal calcifications similar to PTC nodal metastasis.[22,45]

Parathyroid adenomas often are hypoechoic, solid, and show peripheral vascularity on US[13,45] and can mimic level VI PTC nodal metastasis (**Fig. 17**).

Cervical schwannomas (**Fig. 18**) and neurofibromas usually are found in the posterior triangle and within the carotid sheath and can be mistaken

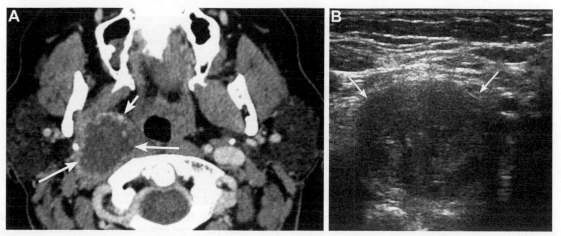

Fig. 18. (*A*) Axial CECT image in a 61-year-old woman at the level of the oropharynx shows a peripherally enhancing and centrally hypodense mass (*long arrows*) in the upper carotid space with anteromedial displacement of the distal ICA (*small arrow*). Schwannoma was favored given the clinical findings. (*B*) GSU of the right carotid space vagal Schwannoma reveals a solid hypoechoic avascular mass (*arrows*) without a hilum that can mimic right level IIA or LRN metastasis.

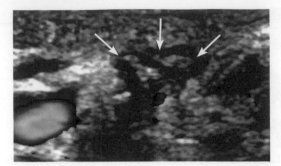

Fig. 19. A GSUD in a 78-year-old man status post–left lateral neck dissection for melanoma 14 months prior, demonstrates a 1-cm hypoechoic left inferior neck nodule (*arrows*) with a triangular configuration with central foci of hyperechogenicity which can mimic PTC nodal metastasis. US-guided FNA = granulation tissue.

for pathologic lymph nodes because of overlapping features, such as cystic changes and irregular vascularity.[22,45] A distinguishing imaging feature of both schwannomas and neurofibromas is the presence of continuity with an adjacent nerve.[22] Along with the posttraumatic neuroma, biopsy of these lesions can result in sharp radiating pain.[45]

Suture granulomas (see **Fig. 19**) are benign inflammatory lesions that may result after surgery and can mimic recurrent malignancy in the thyroid bed because both may show irregular shape, heterogeneous echotexture, variable echogenicity, and internal echogenic foci.[46]

Traumatic neuromas occur in up to 2.7% of neck dissections and can mimic recurrent

lymphadenopathy from thyroid cancer, because both can present on US as a hypoechoic mass with a central area of hyperechogenicity.[47]

Chylous cysts or lymphocele (**Fig. 20**) is a rare complication of injury to the cervical thoracic duct that may occur in neck dissections.[48] Lymphoceles usually are located beneath the SCM and lateral to the carotid sheath and can therefore be confused with a cystic PTC level IV metastasis. Typical imaging features of a lymphocele include a circumscribed cyst with fluid attenuation, which lacks enhancement, nodularity, or internal septations.[48]

Posterior neck nodes can hypertrophy following ipsilateral selective neck dissection with a rounded hypoechoic appearance (see **Fig. 15**). The presence of disorganized vascularity, cystic change, or calcification, however, raises concern for metastasis.

SUMMARY

A comprehensive understanding of sonographic and CECT imaging features of malignant lymph nodes is important for preoperative staging and post-treatment surveillance. Nodal calcification, cystic change, and the presence of disorganized vasculature on GSUD or avid enhancement on CECT are concerning for metastasis. LC nodes with suspicious imaging features can be interrogated with US-guided FNA, and Tg test of the FNA sample can increase sensitivity when cytology is nondiagnostic or discordant with imaging. Furthermore, reactive, inflammatory, granulomatous, or postsurgical lesions as well as various benign tumors can mimic nodal metastasis.

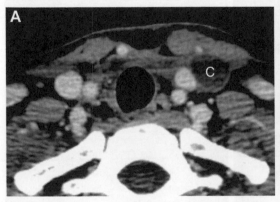
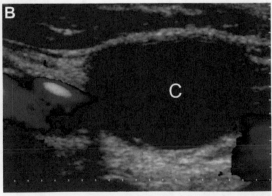

Fig. 20. (*A*) A 31-year-old woman with recurrent PTC treated with left level IV and right level VI lymph node dissection 11 months prior. Axial CECT shows a 2-cm cystic lesion (*C*) in the left lower neck located lateral to the carotid sheath and just proximal to the confluence of the IJV and the subclavian. There is fluid attenuation (hounsfield units 11) without enhancement, nodularity, or septations. (*B*) Concurrent GSUD shows an anechoic cyst (*C*) with increased through transmission and no associated soft tissue nodularity or vascular flow. US-guided FNA demonstrated milky fluid without malignant cells on cytology, and chylocele was identified at surgery performed for other known metastasis.

CLINICS CARE POINTS

- Normal LN are typically oval, with a peripheral cortex hypoechoic to strap muscle, with a central echogenic hilum, and with central hilar vascularity.
- Normal nodes lack calcifications, cystic change, and necrosis.
- Cystic change, intranodal calcification, rounded configuration, and abnormal nodal vascularity are highly specific but relatively insensitive for PTC nodal metastasis.
- Absence of a central echogenic hilum is highly sensitive, although less specific for LN metastasis secondary to PTC.

DISCLOSURE

The authors have nothing to disclose.

REFERENCES

1. Hirokawa M, Ito Y, Kuma S, et al. Nodal metastasis in well-differentiated follicular carcinoma of the thyroid: Its incidence and clinical significance. Oncol Lett 2010;1(5):873–6.
2. Hoang JK, Branstetter BF, Gafton AR, et al. Imaging of thyroid carcinoma with CT and MRI: approaches to common scenarios. Cancer Imaging 2013;13(1):128–39.
3. Suh CH, Baek JH, Choi YJ, et al. Performance of CT in the preoperative diagnosis of cervical lymph node metastasis in patients with papillary thyroid cancer: a systematic review and meta-analysis. AJNR Am J Neuroradiol 2017;38(1):154–61.
4. Haugen BR, Alexander EK, Bible KC, et al. 2015 2015 American Thyroid Association Management Guidelines for Adult Patients with Thyroid Nodules and Differentiated Thyroid Cancer: The American Thyroid Association Guidelines Task Force on Thyroid Nodules and Differentiated Thyroid Cancer. Thyroid 2016;26(1):1–133.
5. Harries V, McGill M, Tuttle RM, et al. Management of retropharyngeal lymph node metastases in differentiated thyroid carcinoma. Thyroid 2020;30(5):688–95.
6. Kim JH, Choi KY, Lee SH, et al. The value of CT, MRI, and PET-CT in detecting retropharyngeal lymph node metastasis of head and neck squamous cell carcinoma. BMC Med Imaging 2020;20(1):88.
7. Yeh MW, Bauer AJ, Bernet VA, et al. American Thyroid Association statement on preoperative imaging for thyroid cancer surgery. Thyroid 2015;25(1):3–14.
8. Langer JE, Mandel SJ. Sonographic imaging of cervical lymph nodes in patients with thyroid cancer. Neuroimaging Clin N Am 2008;18(3):479–viii. vii-viii.
9. Som PM, Curtin HD, Mancuso AA. Imaging-based nodal classification for evaluation of neck metastatic adenopathy. AJR Am J Roentgenol 2000;174(3):837–44.
10. Kouvaraki MA, Shapiro SE, Fornage BD, et al. Role of preoperative ultrasonography in the surgical management of patients with thyroid cancer. Surgery 2003;134(6):946–55 [discussion: 954–5].
11. Ahmed S, Ghazarian MP, Cabanillas ME, et al. Imaging of Anaplastic Thyroid Carcinoma. AJNR Am J Neuroradiol 2018;39(3):547–51.
12. Ying M, Ahuja A. Sonography of neck lymph nodes. part i: normal lymph nodes. Clin Radiol 2003;58(5):351–8.
13. Machado MR, Tavares MR, Buchpiguel CA, et al. Ultrasonographic evaluation of cervical lymph nodes in thyroid cancer. Otolaryngol Head Neck Surg 2017;156(2):263–71.
14. Sohn YM, Kwak JY, Kim EK, et al. Diagnostic approach for evaluation of lymph node metastasis from thyroid cancer using ultrasound and fine-needle aspiration biopsy. AJR Am J Roentgenol 2010;194(1):38–43.
15. Wunderbaldinger P, Harisinghani MG, Hahn PF, et al. Cystic lymph node metastases in papillary thyroid carcinoma. AJR Am J Roentgenol 2002;178(3):693–7.
16. Leboulleux S, Girard E, Rose M, et al. Ultrasound criteria of malignancy for cervical lymph nodes in patients followed up for differentiated thyroid cancer. J Clin Endocrinol Metab 2007;92(9):3590–4.
17. Rosário PWS, de Faria S, Bicalho L, et al. Ultrasonographic differentiation between metastatic and benign lymph nodes in patients with papillary thyroid carcinoma. J Ultrasound Med 2005;24(10):1385–9.
18. Shin LK, Olcott EW, Jeffrey RB, et al. Sonographic evaluation of cervical lymph nodes in papillary thyroid cancer. Ultrasound Q 2013;29(1):25–32.
19. Napolitano G, Romeo A, Vallone G, et al. How the preoperative ultrasound examination and BFI of the cervical lymph nodes modify the therapeutic treatment in patients with papillary thyroid cancer. BMC Surg 2013;13(Suppl 2):S52.
20. Ahuja A, Ying M. Sonography of neck lymph nodes. Part II: abnormal lymph nodes. Clin Radiol 2003;58(5):359–66.
21. Jeon SJ, Kim E, Park JS, et al. Diagnostic benefit of thyroglobulin measurement in fine-needle aspiration for diagnosing metastatic cervical lymph nodes from papillary thyroid cancer: correlations with US features. Korean J Radiol 2009;10(2):106–11.
22. Gritzmann N, Hollerweger A, Macheiner P, et al. Sonography of soft tissue masses of the neck. J Clin Ultrasound 2002;30(6):356–73.

23. Lyshchik A, Higashi T, Asato R, et al. Cervical lymph node metastases: diagnosis at sonoelastography–initial experience. Radiology 2007;243(1):258–67.

24. Kim DW, Choo HJ, Lee YJ, et al. Sonographic features of cervical lymph nodes after thyroidectomy for papillary thyroid carcinoma. J Ultrasound Med 2013;32(7):1173–80.

25. Haugen BR. 2015 American Thyroid Association Management Guidelines for Adult Patients with Thyroid Nodules and Differentiated Thyroid Cancer: What is new and what has changed? Cancer 2017; 123(3):372–81.

26. Som PM. Detection of metastasis in cervical lymph nodes: CT and MR criteria and differential diagnosis. AJR Am J Roentgenol 1992;158(5):961–9.

27. Hoang JK, Vanka J, Ludwig BJ, et al. Evaluation of Cervical Lymph Nodes in Head and Neck Cancer With CT and MRI: Tips, Traps, and a Systematic Approach. AJR Am J Roentgenol 2013;200(1): W17–25.

28. Araque KA, Gubbi S, Klubo-Gwiezdzinska J. Updates on the Management of Thyroid Cancer. Horm Metab Res 2020;52(8):562–77.

29. Robbins KT, Shaha AR, Medina JE, et al. Consensus statement on the classification and terminology of neck dissection. Arch Otolaryngol Head Neck Surg 2008;134(5):536–8.

30. Kupferman ME, Patterson M, Mandel SJ, et al. Patterns of lateral neck metastasis in papillary thyroid carcinoma. Arch Otolaryngol Head Neck Surg 2004;130(7):857–60.

31. Ha EJ, Baek JH, Lee JH, et al. Core needle biopsy could reduce diagnostic surgery in patients with anaplastic thyroid cancer or thyroid lymphoma. Eur Radiol 2016;26(4):1031–6.

32. Grani G, Fumarola A. Thyroglobulin in lymph node fine-needle aspiration washout: a systematic review and meta-analysis of diagnostic accuracy. J Clin Endocrinol Metab 2014;99(6):1970–82.

33. Vu TH, Kwon M, Ahmed S, et al. Diagnostic Accuracy and Scope of Intraoperative Transoral Ultrasound and Transoral Ultrasound-Guided Fine-Needle Aspiration of Retropharyngeal Masses. AJNR Am J Neuroradiol 2019;40(11):1960–4.

34. Henry BM, Sanna S, Graves MJ, et al. The Non-Recurrent Laryngeal Nerve: a meta-analysis and clinical considerations. PeerJ 2017;5:e3012.

35. Watanabe A, Kawabori S, Osanai H, et al. Preoperative computed tomography diagnosis of non-recurrent inferior laryngeal nerve. Laryngoscope 2001;111(10):1756–9.

36. Giugliano G, Proh M, Gibelli B, et al. Central neck dissection in differentiated thyroid cancer: technical notes. Acta Otorhinolaryngol Ital 2014;34(1):9–14.

37. Tufano RP, Clayman G, Heller KS, et al. Management of recurrent/persistent nodal disease in patients with differentiated thyroid cancer: a critical review of the risks and benefits of surgical intervention versus active surveillance. Thyroid 2015;25(1):15–27.

38. Onaran Y, Terzioğlu T, Oğuz H, et al. Great cervical vein invasion of thyroid carcinoma. Thyroid 1998; 8(1):59–61.

39. Uludag M, Ozel A, Aygün N. The clinical importance of tumor thrombus in internal jugular vein related to papillary thyroid cancer. Surg Case Rep 2019; 2019:1–4.

40. Kobayashi K, Hirokawa M, Yabuta T, et al. Tumor thrombus of thyroid malignancies in veins: importance of detection by ultrasonography. Thyroid 2011;21(5):527–31.

41. Karwowski JK, Jeffrey RB, McDougall IR, et al. Intraoperative ultrasonography improves identification of recurrent thyroid cancer. Surgery 2002;132(6): 924–9.

42. DeGroot LJ, Kaplan EL, McCormick M, et al. Natural history, treatment, and course of papillary thyroid carcinoma. J Clin Endocrinol Metab 1990;71(2): 414–24.

43. Schlumberger M, Berg G, Cohen O, et al. Follow-up of low-risk patients with differentiated thyroid carcinoma: a European perspective. Eur J Endocrinol 2004;150(2):105–12.

44. Frasoldati A, Pesenti M, Gallo M, et al. Diagnosis of neck recurrences in patients with differentiated thyroid carcinoma. Cancer 2003;97(1):90–6.

45. Kobaly K, Mandel SJ, Langer JE. Clinical Review: Thyroid Cancer Mimics on Surveillance Neck Sonography. J Clin Endocrinol Metab 2015;100(2): 371–5.

46. Kim JH, Lee JH, Shong YK, et al. Ultrasound features of suture granulomas in the thyroid bed after thyroidectomy for papillary thyroid carcinoma with an emphasis on their differentiation from locally recurrent thyroid carcinomas. Ultrasound Med Biol 2009;35(9):1452–7.

47. Yabuuchi H, Kuroiwa T, Fukuya T, et al. Traumatic neuroma and recurrent lymphadenopathy after neck dissection: comparison of radiologic features. Radiology 2004;233(2):523–9.

48. Hamilton BE, Nesbit GM, Gross N, et al. Characteristic imaging findings in lymphoceles of the head and neck. AJR Am J Roentgenol 2011;197(6): 1431–5.

Surgical Considerations in Thyroid Cancer
What the Radiologist Needs to Know

Daniel Vinh, MD[a], Mark Zafereo, MD[b],*

KEYWORDS

• Thyroid cancer • Surgery • Ultrasound • CT • Radiographic evaluation

KEY POINTS

- This distinction between anterior (strap) and posterior (tracheoesophageal groove) extrathyroidal extension is very important, as anterior extrathyroidal extension can be more confidently resected en bloc with the thyroid with minimal added morbidity, whereas posterior extrathyroidal extension can be more challenging to completely resect and/or lead to more significant surgical morbidity.
- Well-differentiated thyroid cancers rarely involve the esophageal lumen. Often times, the tumor is adherent to the esophageal musculature, which can be removed by resection of the involved muscularis layer, avoiding esophageal lumen entry.
- Unusual vascular anatomy such as a retroesophageal subclavian artery should be noted, as this is associated with a right-sided nonrecurrent laryngeal nerve. Situs inversus should also be assessed, as this can hint a nonrecurrent laryngeal nerve on the left side.
- Common areas of radiographically apparent but surgically "missed" metastatic thyroid cancer lymph nodes in the central and lateral neck compartments include low-level IV nodes, carotid-vertebral nodes, level VB nodes, subdigastric level II nodes medial to the carotid artery, retropharyngeal lymph nodes, and low paratracheal/superior mediastinal lymph nodes.

INTRODUCTION

Thyroid cancer represents about 2% of global cancers diagnosed annually.[1] The incidence of thyroid cancers has nearly tripled in the United States over the last 40 years, with reported increase from 4.9 to 14.3 cases per 100,000 between 1975 and 2009.[2] Around the world, 586,000 patients were diagnosed with thyroid cancer in 2020, ranking nineth in incidence among cancers.[3] Most of this increasing incidence is attributable to increasing incidental detection of small nodules on imaging and screening.[4,5] Although the incidence has increased dramatically, there has not been a corresponding increase in mortality, with overall mortality stable from 1975 to 2009 at approximately 0.5 deaths per 100,000.[2] Most of the thyroid cancers are papillary thyroid carcinoma (PTC), a differentiated thyroid cancer representing approximately 85% of thyroid cancers. Other differentiated thyroid cancers include follicular thyroid carcinoma (FTC) and Hurthle or oncocytic variant thyroid carcinoma. Less common thyroid cancers include medullary, anaplastic, and other cancers arising within the thyroid but not of thyroid origin, such as lymphoma, sarcoma, and distant metastases. The radiologist interpreting thyroid ultrasound or cross-sectional neck imaging will inevitably encounter thyroid carcinoma, and the radiographic assessment serves a vital role in the ultimate management. The diagnosis of thyroid carcinoma is usually confirmed preoperatively with the use of fine-needle aspiration or core needle biopsy in candidate thyroid nodules.[6]

a Department of Otolaryngology - Head and Neck Surgery, Baylor College of Medicine, One Baylor Plaza, Houston, TX 77030, USA; b Department of Otolaryngology - Head and Neck Surgery, MD Anderson Cancer Center, 1515 Holcombe Boulevard, Houston, TX 77030, USA
* Corresponding author.
E-mail address: MZafereo@mdanderson.org

Neuroimag Clin N Am 31 (2021) 327–335
https://doi.org/10.1016/j.nic.2021.04.010
1052-5149/21/© 2021 Elsevier Inc. All rights reserved.

ANATOMY FOR THE RADIOLOGIST

The thyroid gland is a butterfly-shaped organ situated on the midline trachea centered just inferior to the cricoid cartilage. It has 2 lobes connected by an isthmus that may contain a pyramidal lobe in approximately 20% of patients.[7] The thyroid gland lies within the visceral space of the neck, which is surrounded by a layer of thyroid capsule and visceral fascia. Laterally, these 2 fascial layers fuse and insert into the lateral trachea to form a suspensory ligament, known as Berry ligament. The arterial blood supply comes from paired superior thyroid arteries off the external branch of the carotid artery as well as paired inferior thyroid arteries originating from the thyrocervical trunk. The blood supply to the parathyroids is typically from the inferior thyroid arteries. Occasionally, there is a thyroid ima artery that supplies the thyroid isthmus directly from the brachiocephalic trunk. Venous drainage is from paired superior and inferior thyroid veins that drain into the internal jugular and brachiocephalic veins, respectively. There is also a middle thyroid vein that drains into the internal jugular veins. Situated along the posterior surface of the thyroid are 2 superior and 2 inferior parathyroid glands, responsible for maintaining calcium homeostasis. Normal parathyroid glands are typically not readily apparent radiographically, although occasionally normal parathyroid glands can be appreciated on ultrasound.

The recurrent laryngeal nerves are intimately associated with the thyroid gland. They are branches of the vagus nerve and serve the vital role of innervating the majority motor function of the larynx. The left nerve descends into the chest through the carotid sheath, wraps around the ligamentum arteriosum of the aortic arch, and then ascends back into the neck along the tracheoesophageal groove. The right nerve likewise descends into the chest and wraps around the subclavian artery on the right and rises back into the neck in a more lateral to medial trajectory. The right recurrent laryngeal nerve courses more superficially in the right central compartment than the left nerve, and therefore lymph nodes are commonly encountered surgically deep to the right recurrent laryngeal nerve. This location deep to the right recurrent laryngeal nerve can be a common location for missed lymph nodes during a right central compartment dissection. On the other hand, the left nerve has a straighter and deeper course into the cricothyroid joint, and therefore there are rarely lymph nodes deep to the left recurrent laryngeal nerve. Infrequently, the recurrent laryngeal nerve may take a nonrecurrent course and is almost exclusively on the right side. The estimated prevalence is about 0.7% and is associated with an aberrant right subclavian artery in approximately 86.7% of cases[8] or in patients with situs inversus. Preoperative awareness of an aberrant subclavian artery and resultant nonrecurrent right laryngeal nerve can reduce the risk of iatrogenic injury.

The neck anatomy relevant for the radiologist includes the entire anterior neck with an appreciation for adjacent structures and lymphatic drainage pathways of the thyroid (Fig 1). The neck is divided into different lymphatic zones. Level IA, or the submental triangle, is bounded by the anterior bellies of the digastric muscle, the mylohyoid muscle, and the superficial cervical fascia. Level IB is bound by the mylohyoid, the anterior and posterior bellies of the digastric, and the mandible. Level II is bound the SCM muscle, the skull base, the floor of the neck including splenius capitis and levator scapulae, and the hyoid bone. It is further divided into level IIA, superficial and inferior to the spinal accessory nerve, and level IIB, which is deep and superior to the nerve. Level III includes contents along the jugular chain from the hyoid to the cricoid. Level IV includes contents from the cricoid to the clavicle. Level V lymph nodes are the posterior cervical nodes that lie posterior to the posterior border of the SCM muscle and anterior to the trapezius muscle. This group is further divided into level Va superior to the omohyoid muscle and level Vb inferior to the omohyoid muscle. Level VI represent the central compartment lymph nodes that are bound by the cricoid superiorly, the innominate artery inferiorly, and bilateral common carotid arteries laterally. Level VII represents the superior mediastinal lymph nodes. When commenting on lymphadenopathy, detailing the relationship of the nodes to the defined levels as well as to major anatomic structures in the neck aids with surgical planning.

PAPILLARY THYROID CANCER

Papillary thyroid cancer is the most common type of thyroid cancer and is also the main subtype of cancer contributing to the overall growth of thyroid cancer. A SEER database study analyzing the incidence in the United States from 1973 to 2004 found that there has been a 65% to 126% increase in the incidence of PTC, representing 78.6% of all primary thyroid cancer diagnoses.[9] The cause of this increase has been debated, with most arguing that it represents more detection of tumor associated with increased utilization of imaging and a minority suggesting that it could represent a change in environmental exposures such as diagnostic

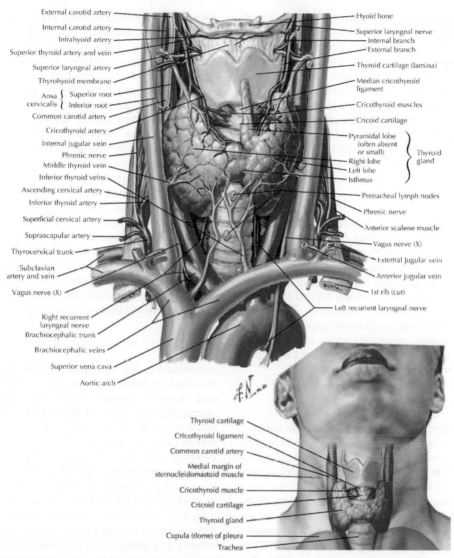

External carotid artery
Internal carotid artery
Infrahyoid artery
Superior thyroid artery and vein
Superior laryngeal artery
Thyrohyoid membrane
Ansa { Superior root
cervicalis { Inferior root
Common carotid artery
Cricothyroid artery
Internal jugular vein
Phrenic nerve
Middle thyroid vein
Inferior thyroid veins
Ascending cervical artery
Inferior thyroid artery
Superficial cervical artery
Suprascapular artery
Thyrocervical trunk
Subclavian artery and vein
Vagus nerve (X)
Right recurrent laryngeal nerve
Brachiocephalic trunk
Brachiocephalic veins
Superior vena cava
Aortic arch

Hyoid bone
Superior laryngeal nerve
Internal branch
External branch
Thyroid cartilage (lamina)
Median cricothyroid ligament
Cricothyroid muscles
Cricoid cartilage
Pyramidal lobe (often absent or small) }
Right lobe } Thyroid gland
Left lobe
Isthmus
Pretracheal lymph nodes
Phrenic nerve
Anterior scalene muscle
Vagus nerve (X)
External jugular vein
Anterior jugular vein
1st rib (cut)
Left recurrent laryngeal nerve

Thyroid cartilage
Cricothyroid ligament
Common carotid artery
Medial margin of sternocleidomastoid muscle
Cricothyroid muscle
Cricoid cartilage
Thyroid gland
Cupula (dome) of pleura
Trachea

Fig. 1. Thyroid gland—anterior view. (*From* Netter's Surgical Anatomy and Approaches. Thyroidectomy and Parathyroidectomy Siperstein, Allan; Benay, Cassandre. Published December 31, 2020. Pages 21-34.)

radiographs.[2,9] The overall prognosis of PTC remains excellent, with an estimated 20-year cancer-specific survival rate of 97%.[5]

Overall, papillary thyroid cancer remains relatively well differentiated, oftentimes with the ability to secrete thyroglobulin and sometimes even produce thyroid hormone. These tumors, therefore, respond to thyroid stimulating hormone suppression, a tactic that is often used in the postoperative setting for higher risk tumors. Classic histopathologic findings include psammoma bodies and papillary fronds with follicular components. The nuclei have an appearance often called "Orphan-Annie" eyes, which reflects a relative clearing within the nuclei.

Although papillary thyroid cancer overall has excellent overall survival, aggressive subtypes

have been identified, including diffuse sclerosing, tall cell or columnar cell variant, and insular thyroid cancer.[10] Diffuse sclerosing is characterized by stromal fibrosis, lymphoid infiltrates, abundant psammoma bodies, and squamous metaplasia and is estimated to account for 2% to 6% of PTC, most commonly seen in children and young adults. The tall-cell variant is characterized by cells having the nuclear features of PTC but with cell body heights 2 to 3 times taller than their width, accounting for about 5% of PTC. A study by Kazaure and colleagues in 2012 found that compared with classic PTC, diffuse sclerosing variant and tall-cell variant had higher rates of aggressive tumor behavior including extrathyroidal extension, multifocality, and nodal and distant metastases.[11]

Another subtype of PTC is the follicular variant of PTC (FVPTC), with cells showing nuclear features typical of PTC but in a growth pattern of neoplastic follicles rather than papillae.[12] FVPTC can be characterized either as encapsulated (EFVPTC) or as non-encapsulated. The treatment of EFVPTC is controversial, as the diagnosis is based on characteristic nuclei and not evidence of invasion.[12] Overall survival for EFVPTC is extremely favorable, leading some to argue that EFPTC is being overtreated with surgery,[13] and along those lines EFVPTC has recently been renamed as noninvasive follicular thyroid neoplasm with papillary-like nuclear features.[14]

Thyroid lobectomy is generally performed for PTC's less than 4 cm without gross extrathyroidal extension and without radiographically apparent lymph node metastases. Even when central compartment lymph node metastases are present, thyroid lobectomy and unilateral central compartment dissection can be considered. However, with significant radiographically apparent lymph node metastases, significant gross extrathyroidal extension, and/or tumors greater than 4 cm, total thyroidectomy is typically recommended.

FOLLICULAR THYROID CARCINOMA

Follicular thyroid carcinoma (FTC) is the second most common well-differentiated thyroid carcinoma, representing approximately 10% of thyroid cancers. Most FTC are encapsulated solid tumors that are macroscopically indistinguishable from minimally invasive FTC. The histopathologic diagnosis of FTC requires capsular and/or vascular invasion. As a result, the diagnosis of FTC is usually made after surgery. As opposed to PTC, FTC is usually not multifocal. In contrast to PTC, the rate of nodal metastasis in FTC is extremely low, whereas the rate of distant metastases in FTC is higher than PTC.[15] Although most of the FTC carries an excellent prognosis, the angioinvasive subtype of FTC has higher rates of distant metastases and poorer overall prognosis.[16] Thyroid lobectomy is typically appropriate for minimally invasive follicular thyroid cancer, whereas total thyroidectomy or completion thyroidectomy (and consideration for postoperative radioactive iodine) is generally recommended for widely invasive and angioinvasive FTC.

HURTHLE CELL (ONCOCYTIC VARIANT) CARCINOMA

Hurthle cells are normal cells with abundant mitochondria found within the thyroid, often associated with Hashimoto thyroiditis. Similar to FTC, Hurthle cell carcinomas are diagnosed based on capsular and/or vascular invasion, and therefore the diagnosis of Hurthle cell carcinoma is typically made after surgical removal of the thyroid lobe or gland. A clinically important distinction of these oncocytic variant carcinomas is their lesser ability to take up iodine, making radioactive iodine treatment less effective.[16] In their clinical behavior, Hurthle cell carcinomas have both a propensity for lymph node metastasis (similar to PTC) and distant metastases (similar to FTC). Overall survival seems comparable with follicular carcinoma, with minimally invasive Hurthle cell carcinomas having excellent prognosis, whereas widely invasive and angioinvasive Hurthle cell carcinomas having relatively poorer prognosis.[17] Similar to FTC, thyroid lobectomy is typically appropriate for minimally invasive follicular thyroid cancer, whereas total thyroidectomy (or completion thyroidectomy) is generally recommended for widely invasive and angioinvasive Hurthle cell carcinoma.

MEDULLARY THYROID CANCER

In contrast to the well-differentiated thyroid cancers and anaplastic thyroid cancer, medullary thyroid cancer arises from the parafollicular neuroendocrine cells of the thyroid, which normally function to produce calcitonin. Approximately 20% of medullary thyroid cancers arise in patients with an inherited multiple endocrine neoplasia syndrome. Medullary thyroid cancers have high propensity for lymph node metastases as well as distant metastases (most commonly lung, liver, and bone). Most patients with medullary thyroid cancer are recommended for total thyroidectomy and bilateral elective central compartment lymph node dissection. Lateral neck dissection is typically reserved for patients with radiographically apparent metastatic lateral neck lymph nodes.[18]

ANAPLASTIC THYROID CANCER

Anaplastic thyroid cancer is a rare form of thyroid cancer that usually presents as a rapidly enlarging neck mass. Representing about 1% of thyroid cancers, it is by far the most clinically aggressive thyroid cancer. Patients present with a rapidly growing neck mass with symptoms including hoarseness, dysphagia, and dyspnea. At the time of initial presentation, most patients will have both locoregionally advanced disease as well as distant metastases. On cross-sectional imaging, these tumors typically demonstrate a mixed solid/necrotic morphology ($\sim$80%) with extrathyroidal extension (>90%); invasion into the esophagus (~60%), trachea (~60%), larynx (~30%), and internal jugular vein (~40%); and carotid artery encasement (~40%).[19] Overall survival has historically been very poor with median less than 6-month survival, but newer molecularly based personalized therapies have recently significantly improved survival in these patients.[20–22]

THE SURGICAL APPROACH
Size and Shape of the Primary Tumor

The size of the primary tumor has significant influence on extent of thyroid surgery. Differentiated thyroid carcinomas less than 1 cm are termed microcarcinomas. Most of the microcarcinomas are PTCs, and these microcarcinomas are largely responsible for the overall increased incidence of thyroid carcinoma.[2] Although the surgical approach for these tumors has typically been thyroid lobectomy, accumulating evidence suggests that many of these tumors may safely undergo active surveillance. Long-term active surveillance programs in Japan from 2 separate hospitals demonstrated that only 8% of patients developed size enlargement and only 4% showed novel nodal metastasis after 10 years of active surveillance. Among the relatively small number of patients who ultimately underwent surgery, none developed recurrence or died of their PTC.[23]

In addition to location of the tumor, it can also be helpful to comment on the shape of the tumor especially when commenting on small tumors. As previously mentioned, micro-PTC represents the bulk of the new and expanding diagnoses of thyroid cancer. Recent data from Japan have suggested that observing these micro-PTCs can be a safe and feasible approach. When evaluating these micro-PTCs, it is important to evaluate the potential for invasion into the recurrent laryngeal nerve, so commenting on its relationship to the expected course of the recurrent laryngeal nerve is important. The tumor's relationship to the trachea is also important, with evidence that tumors that make an obtuse angle with the trachea have a higher likelihood of tracheal invasion as opposed to tumors that make an acute angle. Both of these characteristics of the primary tumor can influence the surgeon's decision to proceed with surgery versus active surveillance.[24]

The 2015 American Thyroid Association guidelines recommend total thyroidectomy for differentiated thyroid cancers greater than 4 cm or tumors that are likely to require adjuvant radioactive iodine. The indications for radioactive iodine are constantly evolving; however, high-risk features such as tumors with significant gross extrathyroidal extension are generally accepted as indications for radioactive iodine.[25,26] For tumors greater than 1 cm and less than 4 cm, either a thyroid lobectomy or total thyroidectomy is considered appropriate, depending on other clinical factors and patient preference. Large studies have demonstrated no difference in survival between thyroid lobectomy and total thyroidectomy for these intermediate size tumors,[27,28] and a recent study by Wrenn and colleagues confirmed that total thyroidectomy was associated with greater rates of hypoparathyroidism, operative time, and length of stay.[29] In addition, most of the patients with normothyroid (approximately 75%) who undergo thyroid lobectomy do not require lifelong hormone replacement. On the other hand, total thyroidectomy allows postoperative thyroglobulin monitoring, potential decreased rates of locoregional recurrence, and less long-term risk of a second surgery to remove the contralateral thyroid lobe, given that papillary thyroid cancer has a high incidence of multifocality within the gland.[30–32] Furthermore, adjuvant treatment in the form of radioactive iodine can only be considered if the patient has undergone a total thyroidectomy.

Location of the Primary Tumor and Extrathyroidal Extension

In addition to tumor size, the location of the tumor in relation to the thyroid gland can influence the surgical approach and should be discussed in a thyroid ultrasound or cross-sectional imaging report. The location of the thyroid tumor in relation to the margin of the gland is important, particularly if the tumor is located at the posterior margin of the gland, where it may interface with the recurrent laryngeal nerve.

Extrathyroidal extension grossly invasive into the strap muscles overlying the thyroid constitutes T3 classification, whereas invasion into visceral structures such as the larynx, trachea, or esophagus constitutes T4a classification. There is controversy regarding the prognostic significance of gross strap muscle invasion, with a recent large single-institution study suggesting that although gross strap muscle invasion may influence risk of locoregional recurrence, it may not affect overall or disease-specific survival.[33] This distinction between anterior (strap) and posterior (tracheoesophageal groove) extrathyroidal extension is very important, as anterior extrathyroidal extension can be more confidently resected en bloc with the thyroid with minimal added morbidity, whereas posterior extrathyroidal extension can be more challenging to completely resect and/or lead to more significant surgical morbidity.[33] Therefore, although thyroid lobectomy may still be considered for patients with anterior gross extrathyroidal extension, total thyroidectomy is generally recommended for patients with differentiated thyroid cancer and posterior extrathyroidal extension, as these patients would be more likely to be recommended for postoperative radioactive iodine therapy.[33]

Tumors with posterior extension beyond the thyroid gland into the tracheoesophageal groove threaten the recurrent laryngeal nerves. Patients who have tumor directly invading the nerve can present with dysphonia and dysphagia. In patients with preoperatively functioning nerves (as evaluated by flexible laryngoscopy), the recurrent laryngeal nerves can usually be preserved. However, significantly counseling is given to patients with gross posterior extrathyroidal extension of disease into the tracheoesophageal groove, if sacrifice of the recurrent laryngeal nerve is necessary, with resultant sequelae on voicing and swallowing. For patients with possible bilateral recurrent laryngeal nerve involvement, the patient must be counseled on the possibility of bilateral recurrent laryngeal nerve injury or sacrifice, potentially necessitating a tracheotomy. Imaging features demonstrating posterior extrathyroidal extension are therefore critical for both preoperative surgical planning and patient counseling.

Tumors that have significant substernal extension are most reliably evaluated with cross-sectional imaging. In most of the cases, a benign substernal thyroid can be removed through a traditional transcervical approach. Rarely, a median sternotomy may be required if the tumor extends inferior to the aortic arch.[34] On the other hand, in the setting of thyroid cancer extending substernally, it is very important to assess potential involvement of the innominate vessels, as involvement of the innominate artery or vein may potentially necessitate sternotomy and/or limit surgical options altogether.

Involvement of the Recurrent Laryngeal Nerve

It is difficult to diagnose recurrent laryngeal nerve invasion on imaging. Although MR imaging has been suggested to predict thyroid cancer invasion into the recurrent laryngeal nerve with 94% sensitivity and 82% specificity,[35] most thyroid experts do not consider MR imaging to be particularly reliable or practically useful for differentiating borderline recurrent laryngeal nerve involvement. If a single recurrent laryngeal nerve is encased by tumor and ipsilateral paralysis or paresis is present preoperatively, en bloc resection of the nerve is necessary to completely remove the gross tumor.

If vocal fold movement is normal, the tumor can generally be shaved off the nerve while sparing the recurrent laryngeal nerve so long as all gross disease is removed.[36] In an instance where a differentiated thyroid tumor encases an recurrent laryngeal nerve and the contralateral nerve is already paralyzed, it is generally recommended to shave the tumor off the nerve in order to avoid the devastating consequence of a bilateral recurrent laryngeal nerve paralysis and the need for tracheostomy. With nerve sacrifice, immediate reanastamosis of the nerve is performed when possible.

Invasion into the Larynx or Trachea

Thyroid cancer invasion into the larynx or trachea is vitally important for surgical planning purposes and dramatically alters the surgical approach. Symptoms that suggest airway invasion include hoarseness, hemoptysis, stridor, and dyspnea. Routes of invasion into the larynx include the cricothyroid membrane, direct invasion through the thyroid cartilage, tracheal invasion with superior growth into the subglottic larynx, or extension of disease posterior to the thyroid cartilage into the pyriform sinus. An important initial distinction when evaluating airway involvement is separating submucosal spread of tumor (more common) versus true endoluminal involvement (less common). If there is high enough suspicion for possible endoluminal involvement, a direct laryngoscopy, tracheoscopy, and bronchoscopy can be planned before or at the time of definitive surgical excision. In the absence of endoluminal invasion, the surgeon can consider shaving procedures or partial laryngectomy to remove gross disease. These techniques demonstrate comparable rates of survival and local control when compared with more radical surgery such as total laryngectomy.[37,38] Indications for total laryngectomy include extensive endoluminal involvement resulting in airway obstruction, hemorrhage, or a dysfunctional larynx preoperatively.[37]

When evaluating tumor invasion into the trachea, a similar surgical decision must be made between a shave excision procedure or resection by a sleeve or window approach. Studies have shown that for carefully selected patients with superficial tracheal involvement, shave resection results in comparable rates of local control when compared with resection of trachea.[39] Imaging that suggests deeper tracheal invasion would prompt the surgeon to consider a window resection of the trachea or circumferential en bloc sleeve resection. Commentating on the expected length of diseased trachea can be helpful, as up to 5 to 6 cm of trachea can be resected and reanastamosed without tracheal or laryngeal mobilization maneuvers.[37,40] When laryngotracheal invasion is suspected, the patient should be referred to a tertiary surgical center that has the experience to handle complex airway procedures and reconstruction.[36]

Invasion of the Esophagus

Well-differentiated thyroid cancers rarely involve the esophageal lumen. Often times, the tumor is adherent to the esophageal musculature, which can be removed by resection of the involved muscularis layer, avoiding esophageal lumen entry; this does not require any reconstruction, although oftentimes a muscle flap such as sternocleidomastoid muscle or strap muscle will be rotated over the surgically demuscularized esophagus. When suspicion for endoluminal involvement is high (eg, a patient with significant dysphagia), this can be confirmed with esophagoscopy. When the esophageal lumen is involved, composite resection should be undertaken. Reconstruction can be performed either with a primary tension-free reanastomosis or a myofascial or myocutaneous pedicled flap or free-flap reconstruction.[36]

Evaluation of Surrounding Vasculature

Unusual vascular anatomy such as a retroesophageal subclavian artery should be noted, as this is associated with a right-sided nonrecurrent laryngeal nerve. Situs inversus should also be assessed, as this can hint a nonrecurrent laryngeal nerve on the left side.[15] When there is concern for arterial vascular invasion on imaging, a dedicated computed tomography angiogram or even full conventional angiography may be needed to assess the vasculature. In the event of planned carotid resection, assessment of the Circle of Willis must be undertaken and the surgeon must be prepared for possible vascular reconstruction.

The most common major vascular structure involved is the internal jugular vein. The vein can lose its patency from direct pressure or frank invasion. In this case, it is important to comment on the patency of the contralateral jugular vein. One internal jugular vein can be excised for en bloc resection of tumor without reconstruction if the contralateral jugular vein is patent. If both veins are sacrificed, the surgeon must be prepared for reconstruction, usually with an autologous vein graft, as bilateral internal jugular vein loss is associated with a 2% mortality.[41]

THE EXTENT OF LYMPHADENECTOMY

Regional lymph node metastases are as high as 30% to 40% in papillary thyroid cancers. If there is suspicious radiographically apparent adenopathy within the central compartment or lateral compartments of the neck, the surgeon will generally perform lymphadenectomy of all at-risk lymph nodes within that compartment of the neck. With respect to removal of radiographically apparent lymph node metastases, complete compartmental resection is generally recommended, with "berry-picking" or selective removal of only single or multiple grossly diseased lymph nodes generally discouraged due to high risk for additional microscopic disease in adjacent lymph nodes. For instance, a unilateral metastatic node within the central compartment will generally result in at least an ipsilateral central compartment neck dissection. If there is lateral nodal disease, then a central and lateral neck dissection is generally performed. In the presence of radiographic lateral neck nodal disease, most investigators advocate for neck dissection of levels IIa, III, IV, and Vb.[42,43] Thyroid cancers rarely metastasize to levels I, Va, and IIb, and these levels are typically not dissected unless there is radiographic suggestion of disease in these specific levels. Common areas of radiographically apparent but surgically "missed" metastatic thyroid cancer lymph nodes in the central and lateral neck compartments include low-level IV nodes, carotid-vertebral nodes, level VB nodes, subdigastric level II nodes medial to the carotid artery, retropharyngeal lymph nodes, and low paratracheal/superior mediastinal lymph nodes.[43] Metastatic retropharyngeal lymph nodes that are larger than 1 to 2 cm are typically surgical excised (often in combination with a lateral neck dissection if there is concomitant lateral neck disease), whereas equivocal or subcentimeter retropharyngeal lymph nodes may be observed and/or treated with postoperative radioactive iodine.[44]

Although there is no role for elective lateral neck dissection (ie, no radiographic evidence of lateral neck disease) in patients with papillary thyroid cancer, the role of elective central neck dissection is controversial. American Thyroid Association guidelines suggest prophylactic central neck dissection may be performed for advanced primary tumors.[26] Arguments for elective central neck dissection for patients with advanced primary tumors include improved accuracy of staging, decreased postoperative thyroglobulin levels, and the potential for decreased reoperations in the central neck, with some evidence that it may lead to lower recurrence.[45]

SUMMARY

The radiographic evaluation of thyroid cancer is critical for treatment planning, especially with regard to location and extent of extrathyroidal extension and presence and extent of lymph node metastases. Although ultrasound is the mainstay of radiographic diagnosis of thyroid cancer and evaluation of suspicious lymph nodes, cross-sectional imaging is a critical component of the evaluation of patients with larger tumors, extrathyroidal extension, and/or radiographically apparent lymph node metastases. Unrecognized and/or underappreciated thyroid disease ultimately leads to unnecessary revision surgeries, increased adjuvant therapy, and higher patient morbidity. Communication between the radiologist, surgeon, and other members of the treatment team cannot be overstated. With improved understanding of surgical and treatment considerations, the radiologist can greatly assist the multidisciplinary team in comprehensive and complete surgical management of thyroid disease, which ultimately translates to fewer revision surgeries and less adjuvant therapy for patients.

Clinics Care Points

- This distinction between anterior (strap) and posterior (tracheoesophageal groove) extrathyroidal extension is very important, as anterior extrathyroidal extension can be more confidently resected en bloc with the thyroid with minimal added morbidity, whereas posterior extrathyroidal extension can be more challenging to completely resect and/or lead to more significant surgical morbidity.

- Well-differentiated thyroid cancers rarely involve the esophageal lumen. Often times, the tumor is adherent to the esophageal musculature, which can be removed by resection of the involved muscularis layer, avoiding esophageal lumen entry.

- Unusual vascular anatomy such as a retroesophageal subclavian artery should be noted, as this is associated with a right-sided nonrecurrent laryngeal nerve. Situs inversus should also be assessed, as this can hint a nonrecurrent laryngeal nerve on the left side.

- Common areas of radiographically apparent but surgically "missed" metastatic thyroid cancer lymph nodes in the central and lateral neck compartments include low-level IV nodes, carotid-vertebral nodes, level VB nodes, subdigastric level II nodes medial to the carotid artery, retropharyngeal lymph nodes, and low paratracheal/superior mediastinal lymph nodes.

DISCLOSURE

The authors have nothing to disclose.

REFERENCES

1. Maniakas A, Davies L, Zafereo ME. Thyroid disease around the world. Otolaryngol Clin North Am 2018; 51(3):631–42.
2. Davies L, Welch HG. Current thyroid cancer trends in the United States. JAMA Otolaryngol Head Neck Surg 2014;140(4):317.
3. Sung H, Ferlay J, Siegel RL, et al. Global cancer statistics 2020: GLOBOCAN estimates of incidence and mortality worldwide for 36 cancers in 185 countries. CA Cancer J Clin 2021. https://doi.org/10.3322/caac.21660.
4. La Vecchia C, Malvezzi M, Bosetti C, et al. Thyroid cancer mortality and incidence: A global overview. Int J Cancer 2015;136(9):2187–95.
5. Davies L, Welch HG. Thyroid cancer survival in the United States. Arch Otolaryngol Head Neck Surg 2010;136(5):440.
6. Yim Y, Baek JH. Core needle biopsy in the management of thyroid nodules with an indeterminate fine-needle aspiration report. Gland Surg 2019;8(Suppl 2):S77–85.
7. Mortensen C, Lockyer H, Loveday E. The incidence and morphological features of pyramidal lobe on thyroid ultrasound. Ultrasound 2014;22(4):192–8.
8. Henry BM, Sanna S, Graves MJ, et al. The Non-Recurrent Laryngeal Nerve: a meta-analysis and clinical considerations. PeerJ 2017;5:e3012.
9. Zhu C, Zheng T, Kilfoy BA, et al. A birth cohort analysis of the incidence of papillary thyroid cancer in the United States, 1973–2004. Thyroid 2009; 19(10):1061–6.
10. Roman S, Sosa JA. Aggressive variants of papillary thyroid cancer. Curr Opin Oncol 2013;25(1):33–8.
11. Kazaure HS, Roman SA, Sosa JA. Aggressive variants of papillary thyroid cancer: incidence, characteristics and predictors of survival among 43,738 patients. Ann Surg Oncol 2012;19(6):1874–80.
12. Nikiforov YE, Seethala RR, Tallini G, et al. Nomenclature revision for encapsulated follicular variant of papillary thyroid carcinoma. JAMA Oncol 2016;2(8):1023.
13. Piana S, Frasoldati A, Di Felice E, et al. Encapsulated well-differentiated follicular-patterned thyroid carcinomas do not play a significant role in the fatality rates from thyroid carcinoma. Am J Surg Pathol 2010;34(6):868–72.
14. Haugen BR, Sawka AM, Alexander EK, et al. American Thyroid Association guidelines on the management of thyroid nodules and differentiated thyroid cancer task force review and recommendation on the proposed renaming of encapsulated follicular variant papillary thyroid carcinoma without invasion to. Thyroid 2017;27(4):481–3.

15. Newman JG, Chalian AA, Shaha AR. Surgical approaches in thyroid cancer: what the radiologist needs to know. Neuroimaging Clin N Am 2008; 18(3):491–504, viii.

16. Sobrinho-Simões M, Eloy C, Magalhães J, et al. Follicular thyroid carcinoma. Mod Pathol 2011; 24(S2):S10–8.

17. Bhattacharyya N. Survival and prognosis in hürthle cell carcinoma of the thyroid gland. Arch Otolaryngol Head Neck Surg 2003;129(2):207.

18. Pena I, Clayman GL, Grubbs EG, et al. Management of the lateral neck compartment in patients with sporadic medullary thyroid cancer. Head Neck 2018;40(1):79–85.

19. Ahmed S, Ghazarian MP, Cabanillas ME, et al. Imaging of anaplastic thyroid carcinoma. AJNR Am J Neuroradiol 2018;39(3):547–51.

20. Maniakas A, Dadu R, Busaidy NL, et al. Evaluation of overall survival in patients with anaplastic thyroid carcinoma, 2000-2019. JAMA Oncol 2020;6(9): 1397–404.

21. Wang JR, Zafereo ME, Dadu R, et al. Complete surgical resection following neoadjuvant dabrafenib plus trametinib inBRAFV600E-mutated anaplastic thyroid carcinoma. Thyroid 2019;29(8):1036–43.

22. Cabanillas ME, Ferrarotto R, Garden AS, et al. Neoadjuvant BRAF- and Immune-Directed Therapy for Anaplastic Thyroid Carcinoma. Thyroid 2018;28(7):945–51.

23. Ito Y, Miyauchi A, Oda H. Low-risk papillary microcarcinoma of the thyroid: A review of active surveillance trials. Eur J Surg Oncol 2018;44(3):307–15.

24. Miyauchi A, Ito Y, Oda H. Insights into the management of papillary microcarcinoma of the thyroid. Thyroid 2018;28(1):23–31.

25. Nixon IJ, Shah JP, Zafereo M, et al. The role of radioactive iodine in the management of patients with differentiated thyroid cancer – An oncologic surgical perspective. Eur J Surg Oncol 2020;46(5):754–62.

26. Haugen BR, Alexander EK, Bible KC, et al. 2015 American Thyroid Association Management Guidelines for Adult Patients with Thyroid Nodules and Differentiated Thyroid Cancer: The American Thyroid Association guidelines task force on thyroid nodules and differentiated thyroid cancer. Thyroid 2016;26(1):1–133.

27. Adam MA, Pura J, Gu L, et al. Extent of surgery for papillary thyroid cancer is not associated with survival. Ann Surg 2014;260(4):601–7.

28. Vargas-Pinto S, Romero Arenas MA. Lobectomy compared to total thyroidectomy for low-risk papillary thyroid cancer: a systematic review. J Surg Res 2019;242:244–51.

29. Wrenn SM, Wang TS, Toumi A, et al. Practice patterns for surgical management of low-risk papillary thyroid cancer from 2014 to 2019: A CESQIP analysis. Am J Surg 2020;221(2):448–54.

30. Iacobone M, Jansson S, Barczyński M, et al. Multifocal papillary thyroid carcinoma—a consensus report of the European Society of Endocrine Surgeons (ESES). Langenbecks Arch Surg 2014; 399(2):141–54.

31. Dhir M, McCoy KL, Ohori NP, et al. Correct extent of thyroidectomy is poorly predicted preoperatively by the guidelines of the American Thyroid Association for low and intermediate risk thyroid cancers. Surgery 2018;163(1):81–7.

32. McDow AD, Pitt SC. Extent of surgery for low-risk differentiated thyroid cancer. Surg Clin North Am 2019;99(4):599–610.

33. Amit M, Boonsripitayanon M, Goepfert RP, et al. Extrathyroidal extension: does strap muscle invasion alone influence recurrence and survival in patients with differentiated thyroid cancer? Ann Surg Oncol 2018;25(11):3380–8.

34. Coskun A, Yildirim M, Erkan N. Substernal Goiter: when is a sternotomy required? Int Surg 2014; 99(4):419–25.

35. Takashima S, Takayama F, Wang J, et al. Using MR imaging to predict invasion of the recurrent laryngeal nerve by thyroid carcinoma. AJR Am J Roentgenol 2003;180(3):837–42.

36. Shindo ML, Caruana SM, Kandil E, et al. Management of invasive well-differentiated thyroid cancer: An American head and neck society consensus statement: AHNS consensus statement. Head Neck 2014;36(10):1379–90.

37. Price DL, Wong RJ, Randolph GW. Invasive thyroid cancer: management of the trachea and esophagus. Otolaryngol Clin North Am 2008;41(6):1155–68.

38. McCaffrey TV, Lipton RJ. Thyroid carcinoma invading the upper aerodigestive system. Laryngoscope 1990;100(8):824–30.

39. Nishida T, Nakao K, Hamaji M. Differentiated thyroid carcinoma with airway invasion: Indication for tracheal resection based on the extent of cancer invasion. J Thorac Cardiovasc Surg 1997;114(1):84–92.

40. Tran J, Zafereo M. Segmental tracheal resection (nine rings) and reconstruction for carcinoma showing thymus-like differentiation (CASTLE) of the thyroid. Head Neck 2019;41(9):3478–81.

41. Kamizono K, Ejima M, Taura M, et al. Internal jugular vein reconstruction: application of conventional type A and novel type K methods. J Laryngol Otology 2011;125(6):643–8.

42. Merdad M, Eskander A, Kroeker T, et al. Metastatic papillary thyroid cancer with lateral neck disease: Pattern of spread by level. Head Neck 2013;35(10):1439–42.

43. Tran J, Zafereo M. Lateral neck dissection for papillary thyroid cancer. VideoEndocrinology 2020;7(4). ve.2020.0199.

44. Tran J, Zafereo M. Parapharyngeal dissection for papillary thyroid cancer. VideoEndocrinology 2019; 6(1). ve.2018.0141.

45. Carling T, Udelsman R. Thyroid Cancer. Annu Rev Med 2014;65(1):125–37.

Radioiodine Imaging and Treatment in Thyroid Disorders

Jeena Varghese, MD[a,*], Eric Rohren, MD, PhD[b], Xu Guofan, MD[c]

KEYWORDS

- Thyroid • Hyperthyroidism • Graves disease • Thyroid cancer • Toxic nodule

KEY POINTS

- Radioiodine uptake scan is a functional study. Hence, it can help identify the cause of thyrotoxicosis.
- Thyroid scintigraphy is used to detect focal and/or global abnormalities of the thyroid gland. It correlates the thyroid anatomy with its function.
- Adequate patient preparation is essential before radioactive iodine scan and treatment of thyroid cancer. This includes withholding thyroid hormone for 3 to 4 weeks or using recombinant human thyroid stimulating hormone (TSH; (thyrotropin alfa) to increase TSH and following a low-iodine diet.
- Factors that interfere or hinder appropriate use of radioactive iodine are recent exposure to iodinated contrast, iodine supplements, and certain medications, such as amiodarone, betadine, and antithyroidal medications (propylthiouracil and methimazole).
- Pregnancy and breastfeeding are absolute contraindication for radioactive iodine and scan.

Since its introduction in the 1940s, radioiodine-131 has been successfully used to evaluate and treat patients with benign and malignant thyroid disease.[1] The thyroid's ability to concentrate radioiodine is helpful in delivering radiation dose to the thyroid tissue that can result in cell destruction without exposing the surrounding organs to lethal radiation. Hyperthyroidism as a result of Graves disease or toxic nodule, and differentiated thyroid carcinoma are indications for use of radioactive iodine therapy. Appropriate use of radioactive iodine requires knowledge of the underlying pathophysiology, its advantages, and limitations.

ANATOMY

The thyroid gland is a midline structure in the anterior neck and is divided into 2 symmetric lobes that are connected by the isthmus. There can be several morphologic variations, including asymmetrical lobes, presence of a pyramidal lobe (remnant of the thyroglossal duct), and ectopic thyroid. Because of the path of embryonic decent, thyroid tissue can be found anywhere from the base of the tongue to the diaphragm.[2] The synthesis of thyroid hormone is dependent on the availability of adequate iodine concentration. Na^+/I^- symporter located on the basolateral membrane of the thyroid follicular cells helps with active transport of iodine into the cytoplasm of the thyrocytes. The Na^+/I^- symporter can obtain an iodine concentration of 20- to 50-fold inside the thyroid cells compared with plasma.[3]

PATHOLOGY

Thyrotoxicosis occurs as a result of high levels of thyroid hormones. Treatment varies with the

[a] Endocrine Neoplasia and Hormonal Disorders, The University of Texas MD Anderson Cancer Center, 1400 Pressler Boulevard, FCT12.5000, Houston, TX 77030, USA; [b] Department of Radiology, Baylor College of Medicine, One Baylor Plaza, Houston, TX 77030, USA; [c] Department of Nuclear Medicine, The University of Texas MD Anderson Cancer Center, 1515 Holcombe Boulevard, Houston, TX 77030-4009, USA
* Corresponding author.
E-mail address: jvarghese@mdanderson.org

Neuroimag Clin N Am 31 (2021) 337–344
https://doi.org/10.1016/j.nic.2021.04.003
1052-5149/21/© 2021 Elsevier Inc. All rights reserved.

cause, and hence, accurate diagnosis is essential. Thyrotoxicosis as a result of hyperthyroidism occurs when there is uncontrolled and autonomous secretion of thyroid hormones. Graves disease is the most common cause of hyperthyroidism followed by toxic multinodular goiter and toxic adenoma. Thyrotoxicosis can also result from destruction or inflammation of the thyroid gland releasing preformed thyroid hormone into circulation. The release of thyroid hormones can be caused by viral infections (painful subacute thyroiditis), medications such as lithium, tyrosine kinase inhibitors, and more recently, immune checkpoint inhibitors used to treat various cancers.

Radioiodine scan is a functional study in contrast to ultrasound or computed tomography (CT), which provides structural information. Hence, in addition to history and physical examination, radioiodine scans can help identify the cause of thyrotoxicosis. As hyperthyroidism is associated with increased thyroid hormone production, there is increased iodine metabolism, which can have elevated radioiodine uptake; whereas in thyroiditis, there will be low or zero radioiodine uptake because of the destruction of thyroid cells.[4]

Other rare causes of hyperthyroidism include exogenous thyrotoxicosis, functioning metastatic thyroid cancer, and Struma ovarii. In these cases, there will be low uptake of radioiodine in the area of the thyroid gland. In patients with Struma ovarii and functional thyroid cancer, there is increased production of thyroid hormones from ectopic thyroid tissues in the ovaries, and hence, a whole-body scan may be needed.[5,6]

Differentiated thyroid cancer accounts for more than 90% of thyroid cancers. This type of cancer is often very indolent and is associated with an excellent prognosis. These cancers include papillary thyroid cancer, follicular thyroid cancer, and hurtle cell cancer. A significant majority of these cancers retain many of the physiologic functions of thyroid cells, including the ability to take up iodine. Thus, radioactive iodine is used as adjuvant therapy to treat residual disease or metastatic disease, providing excellent results in terms of reducing disease recurrence or slowing disease progression.[7]

IMAGING PROTOCOLS

The thyroid uptake examination quantitatively measures the global function of the thyroid gland as reflected by the amount of radiopharmaceutical accumulation and evaluates of iodine kinetics. The uptake procedure can be performed independently, or in conjunction with radioiodine thyroid scintigraphy. A small amount of radioactive iodine, typically 100 μCi (3.7 MBq) iodine-123 or 3 to 4 μCi (0.10–0.15 MBq) iodine-131, is used. Administered activity for children should be determined based on body weight and should be as low as reasonably achievable to perform the radioiodine uptake.

The usual time of measurement is approximately 24 hours after radiopharmaceutical administration. In cases of suspected rapid iodine turnover, an additional uptake measurement may also be performed at 4 to 6 hours. The percent uptake should be compared with normal values measured at the same time after radiopharmaceutical administration. The patient should sit or lie with neck extended. An open-faced collimated detector probe should be directed at the neck, with the crystal usually no more than 20 to 30 cm away.

Thyroid scintigraphy is used to detect focal and/or global abnormalities of the thyroid gland. It correlates the thyroid anatomy with its function and identifies aberrant or metastatic functioning thyroid tissue or residual normal tissue after therapy. Imaging typically includes one or more planar images of the thyroid gland. Radiopharmaceuticals used for imaging include Tc-99m sodium pertechnetate, iodide-123 sodium iodide, or iodide-131 sodium iodide.

Tc-99m pertechnetate is administered intravenously and localizes intracellularly via the sodium/iodide symporter protein. Pertechnetate is not, however, organified within the thyroid and can wash out over time. Imaging can be performed as early as 15 to 30 minutes after administration. Tc-99m pertechnetate is the preferred agent for evaluating congenital hypothyroidism in neonates because of its high-photon flux and lower thyroid radiation exposure. Administered dose for children should be as low as reasonably achievable, with a typical activity range of 2.0 to 5.0 mCi (74–185 MBq) using a reduced adult activity range.

The preferred radiopharmaceutical for thyroid scintigraphy is iodine-123 sodium iodide, given orally, with administered activity of 200 to 400 μCi (7.4–14.8 MBq). With iodine-123, imaging can be obtained as early as 3 to 4 hours or up to 24 hours after administration. Diagnostic-quality images can be obtained as long as 36 hours after administration. Radioiodine is taken up in the thyroid tissues via the sodium/iodide symporter and is organified within the gland. The relatively short half-life and gamma emissions of iodide-123 keep the dose to the thyroid gland low. Use of iodine-131 for imaging is possible but is often avoided because of its much greater radiation dose to the thyroid as a result of longer half-life, along with beta and gamma decay pathways.

When planar imaging is performed, radioactive sources or lead markers may be used to identify anatomic landmarks, such as the sternal notch and thyroid cartilage. The location of palpable nodules should be confirmed with a radioactive point source or lead marker image for anatomic correlation.

The patient should be placed in a supine position, with the neck comfortably extended. When indicated, the physician should palpate the thyroid gland while the patient is in the imaging position as well as when the patient is upright.

Normally, a gamma camera equipped with a pinhole collimator is used. Collimator choice should be appropriate to the radiopharmaceutical used. Images are acquired in the anterior and often both anterior oblique projections for a minimum of 100,000 counts or 8 minutes. There will be significant geometric distortion with the pinhole collimator. Additional views with a parallel-hole collimator may be useful to search for ectopic tissue or estimating thyroid size.

WHOLE-BODY IODINE SCAN FOR THYROID CARCINOMA

Whole-body radioiodine scanning is usually performed for the diagnosis of recurrent thyroid carcinoma. In these patients, the thyroid gland will have been previously resected surgically, and the expectation is that no residual iodine-accumulating tissues will be present in the thyroid bed. Elsewhere in the body, it is expected that no abnormal radioiodine accumulation should occur outside the normal, physiologic pattern. Metastatic disease from thyroid origin, provided the tissue remains differentiated with ability to accumulate radioiodine, will be visualized on scanning.[8]

Pinhole images of the thyroid bed and parallel hole images of the anterior, posterior, and right and left lateral of the head and neck, chest, or abdomen may improve lesion detection relative to the whole-body scan. In addition, single-photon emission computed tomography (SPECT) imaging could be performed to improve sensitivity and specificity if SPECT-CT imaging is available. A high-energy collimator should be used with an appropriately shielded detection head for iodide-131 imaging.

Whole-body scans are usually performed with 2 to 5 mCi of iodine-123 administered 24 hours before the imaging (Fig. 1). They can also be performed with 1.0 to 5.0 mCi of iodine-131 2 to 4 days before the imaging. In patients who receive radioiodine therapy with iodide-131 at higher doses, it is feasible to perform imaging in the post-therapy setting 3 to 7 days after the therapeutic administration (Fig. 2).

When the patient presents with a history of well-differentiated thyroid cancer that is not iodine avid and has elevated thyroglobulin levels, fluorodeoxyglucose PET-CT scans have been used to evaluate non-iodine-avid metastatic disease.

PATIENT PREPARATION (THYROID HORMONE WITHDRAWAL, THYROTROPIN ALFA USAGE, AND LOW-IODINE DIET)

The concentration of radioiodine in functioning thyroid tissue is affected by many factors. Therefore, the thyroid imaging should be delayed long enough to eliminate the confounding effects of the interfering factors.

In the patient with surgical removal of the thyroid gland, thyroid hormone replacement should be withheld for a time sufficient (typically 3–4 weeks) to render the patient hypothyroidic (serum thyroid stimulating hormone [TSH] level >30 mU/L). The patient should be informed of potential side effects of hypothyroidism. In order to avoid severe symptoms of prolonged hypothyroidism, patients may be maintained on triiodothyronine until 10 to 14 days before administration of the radioiodine.

Thyrotropin alpha stimulation could also be used according to the optimize thyroid imaging according to the established protocol. The recombinant human TSH (rhTSH; thyrotropin alfa) is administered intramuscularly as 2 injections of 0.9 mg on 2 consecutive days with iodide-123 or iodide-131 given the next day following the second dose of thyrotropin alfa injection. TSH, serum thyroglobulin, and antithyroglobulin antibody assays will also be obtained 1 to 3 days before radioiodine administration. rhTSH is particularly useful if the patient cannot have near-total thyroidectomy, in the presence of sufficient functioning tumor to suppress endogenous TSH, or with pituitary insufficiency or isolated TSH deficiency.

The absolute contraindication for radioiodine scan is pregnancy. The lactating breast can concentrate iodine, and hence, breastfeeding women are asked to discard expressed milk for about 48 hours after a scan. However, treatment with radioiodine, particularly if used for thyroid cancer, should be avoided, as it can limit the available iodine, making the treatment suboptimal. The other factors that need to be considered are thyroid medications and recent exposure to iodine, which include iodinated contrast, iodine supplements, and certain medications, such as amiodarone, betadine, thyroid hormones, and antithyroid agents (eg, methimazole, propylthiouracil). Antithyroid medications, such as methimazole and propylthiouracil, should be held for 4 to 5 days before a scan and treatment of hyperthyroidism (Table 1).

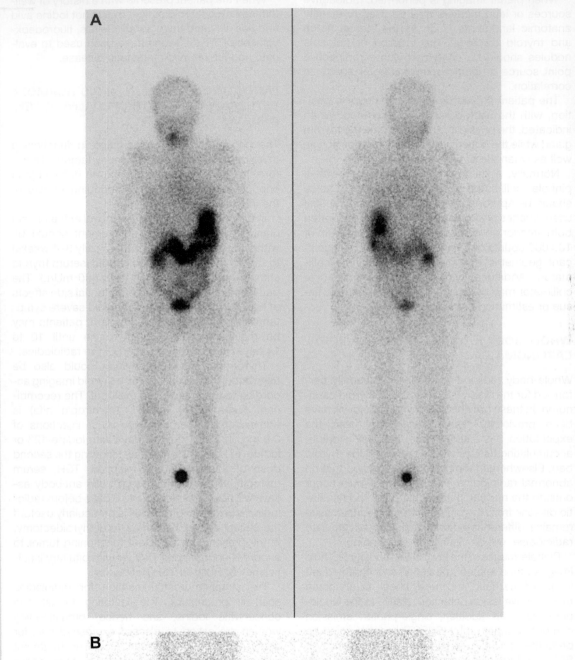

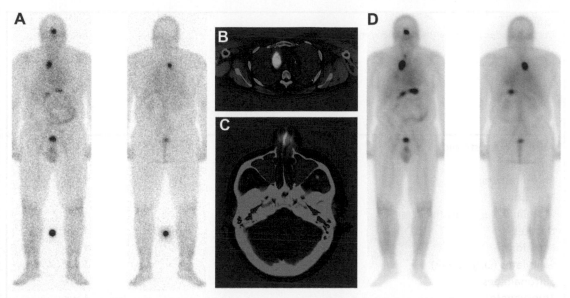

Fig. 2. Metastatic papillary thyroid cancer. A 69-year-old man with metastatic thyroid carcinoma, who had tumor resection and prior radioiodine therapy but with recurrence involving multiple nodes. Whole-body diagnostic iodine-123 scan with 2.2 mCi iodide-124 administered 24 hours before imaging. (A) Anterior and posterior planar images show nodular focus in right superior chest, suggestive of metastatic disease. (B) Fused SPECT/CT axial image shows a large and iodine-avid nodal metastasis in the right lower paratracheal region in the mediastinum. (C) Fused SPECT/CT axial image shows focal avid iodine uptake in the nasal sinus, which represents physiologic activity instead of metastatic disease. (D) The patient was treated with 195 mCi iodide-131. and postablation images were obtained 5 days after therapy. The right chest nodal metastasis shows avid iodine uptake.

A low-iodine diet could increase the sensitivity of thyroid imaging scan and improve the efficacy of iodine-131 ablation. Typically, a low-iodine diet is required at least 2 weeks before radioiodine administration and needs to continue several days during imaging and radioiodine therapy.[9] In the scenario to evaluate for hyperthyroidism, there is a more rapid clearance of iodine. Therefore, successful imaging can often be obtained sooner than the above recommendation. Under very specific circumstances (eg, to determine if a nodule is autonomous), a low-iodine diet may not be necessary.

IMAGING FINDINGS

The radiologist or nuclear medicine physician should correlate the examination with relevant clinical data (eg, thyroid function tests, the presence of clinically palpable neck masses, and potentially interfering substances, such as iodinated radiographic contrast media and medications, vitamins, and health foods containing large amounts of iodine). In addition, correlation with other radiographic modalities, such as ultrasonography, CT, MR Imaging, chest radiography, or other radionuclide imaging studies may also be helpful. Adherence to this guideline should maximize the probability of detecting and characterizing abnormalities of thyroid anatomy and function.

An adequate physical examination and history should be obtained. The presence of palpable tissue in the neck should be defined for correlation with the scintigraphic findings. Special attention should be paid to the precise placement of markers on anatomic landmarks.

For appropriate interpretation of anterior thyroid bed findings, it is necessary to be certain of the location of the nose and/or mouth, thyroid cartilage, and sternal notch in the neck. For whole-body imaging, other landmarks may be important,

Fig. 1. (A) Thyroid scintigraphy and whole-body scan for thyroid cancer with iodide-123 24 hours before the imaging and preparation with rhTSH stimulation. A 26-year-old woman with metastatic papillary thyroid cancer treated with surgery and radioactive iodine. No focal abnormal radiotracer uptake is seen within the neck to indicate iodine-avid recurrent thyroid cancer. (B) Similarly, no abnormal iodine avidity is present within the lungs or elsewhere on the scan to indicate iodine-avid thyroid cancer. Prominent physiologic activity is seen within the bowel and bladder. Uptake in the neck at 24 hours after iodine-123 administration is calculated to be 0.1%.

Table 1
Compounds that may decrease thyroid iodine uptake

Medication	Time (to Wait After Medication is Discontinued)
Adrenocorticosteroids	1 wk
Bromides	1 wk
Phenylbutazone	1 wk
Mercurials	1 wk
Methimazole, propylthiouracil	1 wk
Nitrates	1 wk
Perchlorate	1 wk
Salicylates (large doses)	1 wk
Sulfonamides	1 wk
Thiocyanate	1 wk
Triiodothyronine (liothyronine sodium)	2–3 wk
Thyroid extract	4 wk
Iodine solution (Lugol or saturated solution of potassium iodide) weeks, iodine-containing antiseptics, kelp	4 wk
Some cough medicines and vitamin	4 wk
Intravenous contrast agents	1–2 mo
Oil-based iodinated contrast agents	3–6 mo
Amiodarone	3–6 mo

Adapted from ACR-SNM-SPR practice guidelines for the performance of thyroid scintigraphy and uptake measurements.

such as costal margins, xyphoid process, pubic symphysis, iliac crests, or the location of the spine. In addition to the scintigraphic images with markers, duplicate images should be obtained without the markers to avoid interference with areas of uptake adjacent to the markers.

The report should include a qualitative estimate of the size, activity, and location of any areas of uptake that correspond to any functioning normal or abnormal thyroid tissue. Particular attention should be paid to activity in the thyroid bed. Scan images cannot differentiate residual normal thyroid tissue (eg, thyroid remnants) from tumor. Comparison with prior scans can often be useful in defining the significance of localized neck activity. Lateral and oblique views may be useful in separating thyroid bed activity from neighboring lymph node activity. Results of recent thyroglobulin assays may be useful, especially in interpreting negative scintigraphic finding, recognizing that about 20% of patients with thyroid cancer have antibodies to thyroglobulin, which invalidate the serum thyroglobulin measurement.

TREATMENT OF THYROID DISEASE WITH RADIOIODINE

Iodide-131 is a β-emitting radionuclide with a physical half-life of 8.1 days. It has a principal λ-ray of 364 keV, and a principal β-particle with a maximum energy of 0.61 MeV, an average energy of 0.192 MeV, and a mean range in tissue of 0.4 mm.[10] Oral administration of iodide-131 sodium iodine as commonly accepted treatment of thyroid disease has been established for decades.

Common indications for treatment with iodide-131 include benign diseases, such as hyperthyroidism, Graves disease (**Fig. 3**), toxic nodular disease (**Fig. 4**), and malignant thyroid disease, including the differentiated papillary and follicular thyroid cancer. Iodide-131 ablation therapy refers to the use of iodide-131 to eliminate residual normal thyroid tissue detected after thyroidectomy, after residual or recurrent thyroid cancer, and of metastatic disease after near-total thyroidectomy. The goal of therapy for hyperthyroidism is to achieve either a euthyroid state or an iatrogenic hypothyroidism. After the therapy, the patient will achieve the euthyroid state with oral levo-thyroxine. For the large nontoxic nodular goiter, the goal is to reduce thyroid volume to relieve the compression of the goiter on the neck structures.

Iodide-131 ablative treatment of differentiated thyroid cancer is recommended in the postsurgical management of patients with a maximum tumor diameter greater than 1.0 cm or with a maximum tumor diameter less than 1.0 cm in the presence of high-risk features, such as aggressive histology (Hurthle cell, insular, diffuse sclerosing, tall cell, columnar cell, trabecular, solid, and poorly differ-entiated subtypes of papillary carcinoma), lymphatic or vascular invasion, lymph node or distant metastases, multifocal disease, capsular invasion or penetration, perithyroidal soft tissue involvement,[11] or an elevated antithyroglobulin antibody level after thyroidectomy. The treatment of very-low and low-risk thyroid cancers with iodide-131 is controversial, as data suggest no significant improvements in disease-specific sur-vival.[12] However, the recurrence rates may decrease.[13] The treatment choices depend on many factors, including the pathologic condition, location, and size of thyroid cancer. The presence or absence of iodine-accumulating thyroid tissue before ablation should be evaluated by uptake measurement and imaging.

The American Thyroid Association Guideline sug-gests not imaging before iodide-131 therapy.[7] Nu-clear medicine consultants are divided as to the need for thyroid imaging before iodide-131 ablation. Such thyroid scan could identify low but finite fre-quency of significant clinical problems. For example, about 1% of the thyroidectomy is truly total, and there will be no remnant thyroid tissue to be ablated. If the postoperative thyroid remnant remains too large, the usual ablation dose (ranging from 50 to 150 mCi) might cause radiation thyroiditis with sig-nificant neck pain and swelling. If distant metastases are identified in the brain or spinal cord, preradiation corticosteroids are needed to avoid complications caused by radiation-induced swelling. If regional or distant metastases are detected on the preablation scan, larger dosages of radioiodine are usually given at the time of ablation.

In general, higher iodide-131 dose is required for treatment of the more invasive or disseminated thy-roid cancer at the time of therapy or greater risk of metastases or recurrent tumor. For postoperative ablation of thyroid bed remnants, activity in the range of 1.11 to 3.7 GBq (30–100 mCi) is typically prescribed, depending on the radioiodine uptake measurement and amount of residual functioning tissue present. However, the rate of successful remnant ablation in patients who have undergone total or near-total thyroidectomy appears to be not

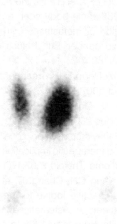

Fig. 3. Graves disease. A 59-year-old woman with hy-perthyroidism. Uptake in the thyroid is calculated to be 34% at 4 hours (normal: 6%–18%); 50% at 24 hours (normal: 10%–35%). Homogeneous radiotracer up-take is seen in the bilateral lobes of thyroid, with the left lobe anatomically larger than the right.

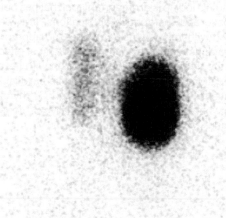

Fig. 4. Autonomous thyroid nodule. A 39-year-old woman with hyperthyroidism and thyroid nodule. Up-take in the thyroid is calculated to be 24.3% at 5 hours (normal: 6%–18% at 4 hours); 30.5% at 24 hours (normal: 10%–35%). A large nodular/ovoid activity in region of left thyroid, with relative loss of uptake in the right thyroid, probably because of suppression from the left thyroid autonomous nodule.

inferior in patients treated with 30 mCi compared with 100 mCi in most studies comparing these activities and particularly in studies achieving the highest successful ablation rates.[7] Patients with advanced local or regional disease may be treated first with surgical debulking and then with iodide-131 and/or external beam radiation. For treatment of distant metastases, an activity of 7.4 GBq (200 mCi) or more is often given. The radiation dose to the bone marrow is typically the limiting factor. An elevated or rising serum thyroglobulin level is a useful indicator of residual or recurrent thyroid cancer in the absence of antithyroglobulin antibodies. It may be an indication for empiric radioiodine therapy, using 5.55 to 7.40 GBq (150–200 mCi), even in the absence of discernible activity on the diagnostic radioiodine scan.

WHAT THE PHYSICIAN NEEDS TO KNOW

The treating physician must explain the procedure, treatment, complications, side effects, therapeutic alternatives, and expected outcome to the patient. Written information must be provided to the patient according to the Nuclear Regulatory Commission (NRC).[14] The treating physician should obtain written informed consent before therapy. The facility must be licensed to receive, store, and handle radioactive iodine, and follow NRC guidelines for patient discharge.

SUMMARY

Radioactive iodine is an important tool that has both diagnostic and therapeutic applications. It is well tolerated with very few risks. When used appropriately, radioactive iodine therapy will be most effective in the treatment of hyperthyroidism with fewer complications. It also can help improve survival in the patient with intermediate- to high-risk thyroid cancer where cancer has spread to the lymph nodes in the neck or other parts of the body.

CLINICS CARE POINTS

- Radioactive iodine scan is a non-invasive imaging used for functional assessment of thyroid disorders and to treat thyroid cancer remnant or distant metastasis.
- It is well tolerated, and pregnancy/breastfeeding are the only absolute contraindication.
- Adequate preparation with low iodine diet and avoidance of interfering medications are needed for optimal results.

DISCLOSURE

J. Varghese, E. Rohren, and X. Guofan have nothing to disclose.

REFERENCES

1. Chapman EM, Evans RD. The treatment of hyperthyroidism with radioactive iodine. J Am Med Assoc 1946;131:86–91.
2. Patel S, Bhatt AA. Thyroglossal duct pathology and mimics. Insights Imaging 2019;10(1):12.
3. Leung A, Pearce EN, Braverman LE. Role of iodine in thyroid physiology. Expert Rev Endocrinol Metab 2010;5(4):593–602.
4. Ross DS, Burch HB, Cooper DS, et al. 2016 American Thyroid Association Guidelines for diagnosis and management of hyperthyroidism and other causes of thyrotoxicosis. Thyroid 2016;26(10):1343–421.
5. Ang LP, Avram AM, Lieberman RW, et al. Struma ovarii with hyperthyroidism. Clin Nucl Med 2017;42(6):475–7.
6. Ober KP, Cowan RJ, Sevier RE, et al. Thyrotoxicosis caused by functioning metastatic thyroid carcinoma. A rare and elusive cause of hyperthyroidism with low radioactive iodine uptake. Clin Nucl Med 1987;12(5):345–8.
7. Haugen BR, Alexander EK, Bible KC, et al. 2015 American Thyroid Association Management Guidelines for adult patients with thyroid nodules and differentiated thyroid cancer: the American Thyroid Association Guidelines Task Force on Thyroid Nodules and Differentiated Thyroid Cancer. Thyroid 2016;26(1):1–133.
8. de Geus-Oei LF, Oei HY, Hennemann G, et al. Sensitivity of 123I whole-body scan and thyroglobulin in the detection of metastases or recurrent differentiated thyroid cancer. Eur J Nucl Med Mol Imaging 2002;29(6):768–74.
9. Iagaru A, McDougall IR. Treatment of thyrotoxicosis. J Nucl Med 2007;48(3):379–89.
10. Eckerman KF. Decay, dosimetry, nuclear medicine. Radioisotopes 2007;43.
11. Pazaitou-Panayiotou K, Capezzone M, Pacini F. Clinical features and therapeutic implication of papillary thyroid microcarcinoma. Thyroid 2007;17(11):1085–92.
12. Sacks W, Fung CH, Chang JT, et al. The effectiveness of radioactive iodine for treatment of low-risk thyroid cancer: a systematic analysis of the peer-reviewed literature from 1966 to April 2008. Thyroid 2010;20(11):1235–45.
13. Jonklaas J, Sarlis NJ, Litofsky D, et al. Outcomes of patients with differentiated thyroid carcinoma following initial therapy. Thyroid 2006;16(12):1229–42.
14. 35.75 S. Release of individuals containing unsealed byproduct material or implants containing byproduct material. January 1, 2011.

PET/Computed Tomography in Thyroid Cancer

Divya Yadav, MD[a], Komal Shah, MD[b], Kylan Naidoo[c],
Devaki Shilpa Sudha Surasi, MD[d,*]

KEYWORDS

- [18]F FDG-PET/CT • PET • Thyroid cancer • DTC • ATC • MTC

KEY POINTS

- PET with fludeoxyglucose F 18 (^{18}F FDG-PET) imaging is primarily considered in patients with high-risk differentiated thyroid cancers with elevated serum thyroglobulin level (>10 ng/mL) and negative radioiodine scintigraphy.
- [18]F FDG-PET may be considered as a part of initial staging in poorly differentiated thyroid cancers, anaplastic thyroid carcinomas, and invasive Hürthle cell carcinomas.
- It can also be used as a prognostic tool in patients with metastatic disease to identify patients at highest risk for rapid disease progression.
- Although ^{18}F-FDG has a limited role in medullary thyroid cancer, ^{68}Ga-DOTATATE and ^{18}F-fluoro-dihydroxyphenylalanine PET can be considered in detecting recurrent disease.

INTRODUCTION

Thyroid cancer is the most common endocrine cancer, and its incidence has markedly increased over the last decade, substantially due to increased detection by the use of highly sensitive diagnostic procedures.[1] Currently, it accounts for approximately 2.0% to 3.0% of all new cancers diagnosed each year in the United States.[2] Based on histology, primary thyroid cancers are commonly classified into papillary thyroid carcinoma (PTC), follicular thyroid carcinoma (FTC), Hürthle cell thyroid carcinoma (HCTC), medullary thyroid carcinoma (MTC), and anaplastic thyroid carcinoma (ATC). Other primary thyroid cancers such as squamous cell carcinoma, mesenchymal tumors, and lymphoma are extremely rare.[3] Each of these histologically classified diseases is biologically and clinically distinct.[4] PTC and FTC are classified as differentiated thyroid cancers (DTCs), which have an excellent prognosis with 10-year survival rates of greater than 95% and 90%, respectively.[1,5] DTC comprises the majority (>90%) of thyroid cancers and has a less than 20% overall risk of relapse. However, recurrence and survival rates of patients with MTC and HCTC are significantly worse, with a disease-specific 10-year survival rate of around 85% to 90%.[6,7] On the contrary, ATC typically occurs in elderly and has very poor outcome with a 5-year survival rate of only around 7%.[8]

According to the guidelines proposed by American Thyroid Association (ATA), European Thyroid Association, National Cancer Comprehensive Network,[9] and other professional associations involved, the treatment of patients with DTC

[a] Department of Radiation Oncology, The University of Texas MD Anderson Cancer Center, 1400 Pressler, FCT 16.6014, Unit 1483, Houston, TX 77030, USA; [b] Department of Neuroradiology, Division of Diagnostic Imaging, The University of Texas MD Anderson Cancer Center, 1400 Pressler, Unit 1482, Houston, TX 77030, USA; [c] Department of Abdominal Imaging, Summer Student Program, Division of Diagnostic Imaging, The University of Texas MD Anderson Cancer Center, 1400 Pressler, FCT 16.6014, Unit 1483, Houston, TX 77030, USA; [d] Department of Nuclear Medicine, Division of Diagnostic Imaging, The University of Texas MD Anderson Cancer Center, 1400 Pressler, FCT 16.6014, Unit 1483, Houston, TX 77030, USA
* Corresponding author.
E-mail address: dssurasi@mdanderson.org

Neuroimag Clin N Am 31 (2021) 345–357
https://doi.org/10.1016/j.nic.2021.04.004

begins with thyroidectomy followed by radioiodine (RAI) therapy or external beam radiation therapy, depending on the histology and tumor stage. Several imaging modalities such as ultrasonography (US), computed tomography (CT), MR imaging, and PET have been advocated in the evaluation of thyroid cancers. PET with fludeoxyglucose F 18 (^{18}F FDG-PET) has emerged as an important diagnostic tool in the management of numerous solid tumors.[10] The aim of this review is to focus on the evolving role of FDG PET/CT in the management of thyroid cancers.

Conventional Imaging

ATA recommends US as the first diagnostic test of choice for evaluating thyroid nodules and for preoperative evaluation of the contralateral lobe and cervical lymph nodes.[11] It is widely available, easy to perform, and can be readily combined with fine-needle aspiration (FNA) biopsy. The Thyroid Imaging Reporting and Data System (TIRADS) uses US features (composition, echogenicity, shape, margin, and echogenic foci)[12] to indicate the risk of malignancy, estimated at 0.3% for TR1, 1.5% for TR2, 4.8% for TR3, 9.1% for TR4, and 35% for TR5[13] (see Harshawn S. Malhi and Edward G Grant article, "Ultrasound of Thyroid Nodules and TIRADS," in this issue for an in-depth description of the TIRADS system). Other modalities such as CT and MR imaging can provide valuable anatomic information about the thyroid and surrounding structures during the initial workup of thyroid cancer. FDG PET is not routinely recommended in the initial workup of DTC.[11] CT has a sensitivity of 80% to 90.6% for detecting cervical metastases,[14] but it may fail to detect pulmonary micrometastases that may be evident on radioiodine scintigraphy.[15]

US of the neck is also the first imaging investigation for suspected thyroid cancer recurrence. If the ultrasound is negative in patients with DTC, radioiodine (^{131}I) whole-body scintigraphy (WBS) is the next investigation for identifying remnant thyroid tissue, distant metastatic disease, and further treatment planning.[11] Diagnostic WBS and thyroglobulin (Tg) levels, either following thyroid hormone withdrawal or recombinant human thyroid-stimulating hormone (Thyrogen), performed 6 to 12 months after adjuvant RAI therapy can be useful in the follow-up of patients with high or intermediate risk (higher risk features) of persistent disease.[11]

Incidental Diffuse and Focal Fludeoxyglucose Thyroid Uptake

Incidental FDG uptake in the thyroid gland has been reported in 1% to 4% of patients undergoing FDG PET for other reasons. Diffuse increased uptake in the thyroid has been reported in 0.6% to 3.3% of patients undergoing FDG PET and commonly represents a benign pathology (ie, chronic lymphocytic thyroiditis).[16] ATA 2015 guidelines suggest that diffuse FDG uptake, in conjunction with US and clinical evidence of chronic lymphocytic thyroiditis, does not require further evaluation.[11] Because FDG PET has routine oncology application in response assessment, it is frequently encountered with radiation-induced and immunotherapy-induced thyroiditis (Fig. 1).[17,18] Interestingly, FDG PET has been proposed to predict the development of immunotherapy-induced thyroiditis with subsequent hypothyroidism even before laboratory testing.[19]

Incidental hypermetabolic thyroid nodules were found in 1% to 2% of FDG PET/CT studies, according to one systematic review of more than 125,000 scans.[20] Further evaluation based on US features and size of the thyroid nodule incidentally detected on PET/CT or CT can help to better stratify the malignancy risk.[21] The risk of malignancy in incidental focal thyroid uptake on PET has been reportedly high (21%–36%).[20,22] Given the indolent nature of most PTCs, the decision to proceed with US and FNA should take any serious patient comorbidities into consideration (Fig. 2). A white paper from the American College of Radiology regarding incidental thyroid nodules also makes this recommendation (Fig. 3).[21]

Evaluation of Thyroid Nodule with Indeterminate Cytology

In case of thyroid nodules with indeterminate cytology, FDG PET/CT has a moderate ability to correctly discriminate malignant from benign lesions.[23] With a high negative predictive value, FDG PET can serve as a rule-out test to reduce unnecessary diagnostic surgeries.[24] It could prevent up to 47% of unnecessary surgeries, leading to lower costs and a modest increase of health-related quality of life.[25] However, the sensitivity and specificity of PET is too low to routinely recommend it for the evaluation of thyroid nodules with indeterminate cytology. In a prospective analysis of 56 nodules with indeterminate cytology, Deandreis and colleagues demonstrated that adding FDG PET findings to neck US provided no diagnostic benefit or improved risk assessment.[26]

Differentiated Thyroid Cancer

FDG PET/CT is primarily considered in patients with high-risk DTC with elevated serum thyroglobulin levels (Tg >10 ng/mL) and a negative ^{131}I-WBS imaging (Fig. 4).[11] In a meta-analysis by Qichang

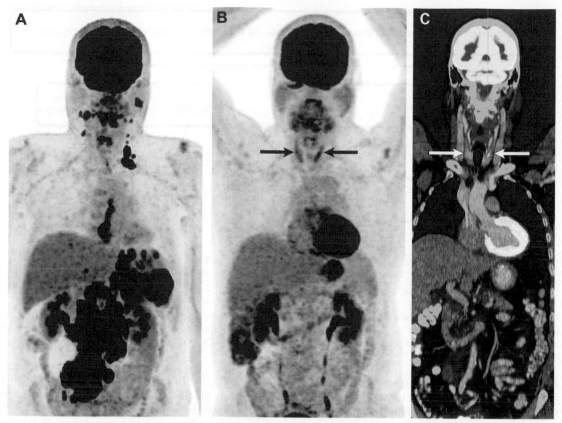

Fig. 1. A 54-year-old man had wide local excision of left calf melanoma. Sentinel lymph node dissection showed inguinal micrometastasis. (A) FDG PET maximum intensity projection (MIP) showed metabolically active adenopathy above and below the diaphragm. After 2 cycles of nivolumab at outside institution for presumed metastatic melanoma, biopsies both above and below the diaphragm revealed follicular lymphoma. The patient was treated with rituximab and lenalidomide. (B) FDG PET MIP at 6 months after scan in (A) showed complete metabolic response. New diffuse, mild uptake in the thyroid gland, with a characteristic butterfly shape (arrows), was in keeping with treatment-induced thyroiditis. (C) Coronal PET/CT fusion images confirm registration of metabolic activity to the thyroid gland.

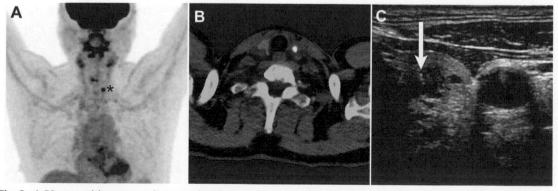

Fig. 2. A 50-year-old man was diagnosed with stage IV non–small cell lung cancer metastatic to bone and adrenal glands 3 years ago. He had systemic therapy with complete metabolic response. (A) FDG PET MIP and (B) Axial FDG PET/CT showed incidental focal activity in the left thyroid lobe with SUV 5.9 (*). The focus was stable from PET/CT 18 months prior. (C) Ultrasound (US) showed 0.8 cm hypoechoic nodule with punctate echogenic foci (arrow). Fine-needle aspiration (FNA) was performed to exclude thyroid metastasis not responding to therapy. Cytology showed papillary thyroid cancer (PTC). No therapy for PTC was planned.

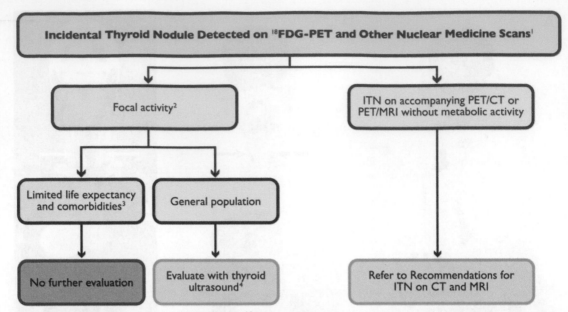

Fig. 3. Incidental thyroid nodule detected on ¹⁸F FDG-PET and other nuclear medicine scans. (*From* Hoang JK, Langer JE, Middleton WD, et al. Managing incidental thyroid nodules detected on imaging: white paper of the ACR Incidental Thyroid Findings Committee. J Am Coll Radiol JACR. 2015;12:143-150; with permission.)

and colleagues, FDG PET/CT was shown to have a high diagnostic accuracy for detection of recurrent and metastatic disease in patients with DTC with thyroglobulin elevation and negative iodine scintigraphy. The results of this analysis showed a sensitivity of 0.86 (95% confidence interval [CI]: 0.79–0.91), a specificity of 0.84 (95% CI: 0.72–0.91), and an area under the curve of 0.91 (95% CI: 0.88–0.93).[27] In another meta-analysis of 25 studies including 789 patients, the sensitivity of FDG PET/CT was 83% (CI 50%–100%) and the specificity was 84% (CI 42%–100%) in non¹³¹I-

avid DTC.[28] FDG PET/CT also showed higher sensitivity (94.3%, CI 87%–97%) when compared with conventional imaging (65.4%, CI 32%–88%) in patients with suspected recurrence of DTC.[29] Moreover, it also exhibits high specificity in detection of metastatic lymph nodes in patients with DTC.[30]

In patients with DTC showing undetectable Tg levels with persistent anti-Tg antibodies, the level of serum Tg cannot be reliably assessed and FDG PET/CT may localize disease in some of these patients.[31] After the first posttreatment WBS

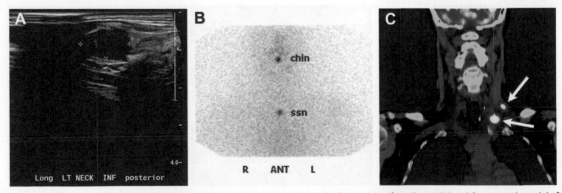

Fig. 4. A 52-year-old woman had total thyroidectomy and neck dissection showing PTC with central and left lateral neck nodal metastases. She was followed with negative radioactive iodine studies at 3 months and 11 months after surgery. One year postoperatively, US in (*A*) showed a suspicious left inferior neck node without discernible hilum. Three weeks later, recombinant human TSH-stimulated ¹³¹I scan (*B*) was again normal. Thyroglobulin level at that time is unknown. (*C*) FDG PET-CT showed metabolically active left inferior neck nodes (*arrows*). Left neck dissection 1 month after (*C*) showed matted left neck nodal metastases from PTC.

performed following RAI remnant ablation or adjuvant therapy, low-risk and intermediate-risk patients (lower risk features) with an undetectable Tg on thyroid hormone with negative anti-Tg antibodies and a negative US do not require routine diagnostic WBS during follow-up. Most well-differentiated thyroid carcinomas are relatively slow growing and can be FDG negative in follow-up. FDG PET/CT can be used in patients in whom DTC cells dedifferentiate, their radioiodine uptake decreases and glucose metabolism increases, described as a RAI-refractory disease.[32] FDG PET/CT can be complementary to ^{131}I-WBS, even in the presence of detectable ^{131}I uptake in metastases, because FDG uptake may be present in neoplastic foci with or without ^{131}I uptake. These patients with FDG-avid metastatic RAI-refractory disease are more likely to develop progressive disease, and FDG PET/CT can provide an early response assessment to systemic therapies, for example, tyrosine kinase inhibitors (Fig. 5).[32,33]

The factors influencing FDG uptake include age, tumor dedifferentiation, larger tumor burden, and to a lesser extent, TSH stimulation.[34,35] FDG uptake on PET in patients with metastatic DTC is a major negative predictive factor for response to RAI treatment and an independent prognostic factor for survival.[36] The maximum standardized uptake value (SUV) and the number of FDG avid lesions were also related to prognosis ($P = .03$ and .009).[36] It can also identify lesions with high FDG uptake that may be more aggressive and should be targeted for therapy or close monitoring. FDG PET/CT imaging also has a significant clinical impact on management. In a study by Larg and colleagues, the treatment strategy was changed in 89.2% cases of positive PET/CT scans in patients with DTC.[37]

Hürthle Cell Thyroid Carcinoma

Hurthle cell thyroid carcinoma is an aggressive histologic subtype of thyroid cancer, with intense FDG uptake and an inability to concentrate [131]I (Fig. 6).[38] With poor ^{131}I concentration, accurate localization of disease using PET is essential,

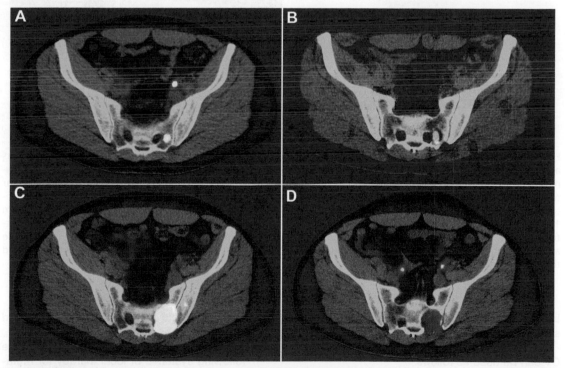

Fig. 5. A 45-year-old man had total thyroidectomy for follicular variant of papillary thyroid cancer, BRAF V600E mutation negative, followed by radioactive iodine ablation. Two years later his thyroglobulin suddenly reached 62 ng/mL and increased to 150 ng/mL 1 month later. (A) Axial FDG PET/CT showed left sacral activity, SUV 5.6, within a small lytic bone lesion. Soon after, biopsy of the left sacrum confirmed metastasis. (B) Three weeks after biopsy, ^{123}I SPECT/CT showed focal activity. [131]I treatment was administered. (C) FDG PET/CT 8 months after radioactive iodine therapy shows dramatic increase in size and activity (SUV 9.2) of left sacral metastasis. The patient underwent proton radiation therapy. (D) Treatment response, SUV 3.7, was seen on FDG PET/CT 21 months after proton radiation.

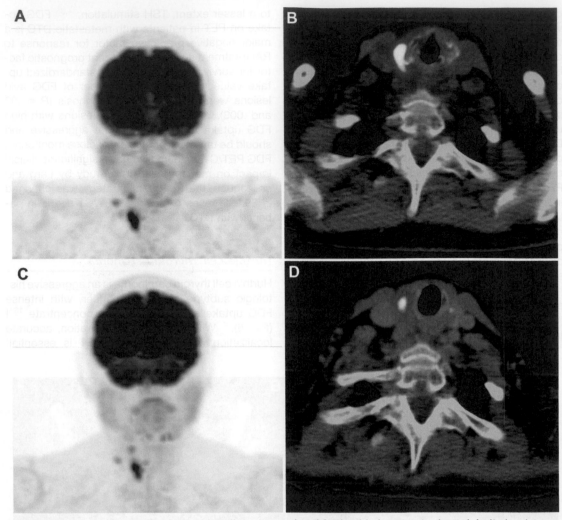

Fig. 6. A 74-year-old woman with Hurthle cell carcinoma (HCC) had mild elevation in thyroglobulin level 4 years after surgery. FDG PET MIP in (A) and axial fused FDG PET/CT in (B) showed suspected recurrence in the right thyroid bed (SUV 18) and in small right neck nodes. Right thyroid bed FNA confirmed recurrent HCC. After molecular testing of the tumor, lenvatinib therapy was started. Pembrolizumab was added 7 months later. FDG PET/CT obtained every 3–4 months after study in (A) and (B) showed stable anatomic appearance with SUV fluctuating from 11 to 20, likely related to immunotherapy. The nodal sites over this time also demonstrated stable size and fluctuating SUV. (C) FDG MIP and (D) axial fused FDG PET/CT obtained 19 months after (A) and (B) show stable anatomic appearance of right thyroid bed recurrence (SUV 11). There was no new evidence of metastasis, and this was interpreted as stable disease.

because appropriate management may provide survival benefit.[39]

ATA 2015 guidelines[11] proposed that FDG PET/CT can be used as follows:

- Part of initial staging in poorly DTCs and invasive Hürthle cell carcinomas, especially those with other evidence of disease on imaging or because of elevated serum Tg levels,
- Prognostic tool in patients with metastatic disease to identify lesions and patients at highest

risk for rapid disease progression and disease-specific mortality, and
- Evaluation of posttreatment response following systemic or local therapy for metastatic or locally invasive disease.

Several studies have reported high sensitivity of FDG PET/CT in HCTC. Lowe and colleagues found that FDG PET/CT had a sensitivity of 92% in 14 scans of 12 patients with HCTC and detected disease not seen on conventional imaging modalities

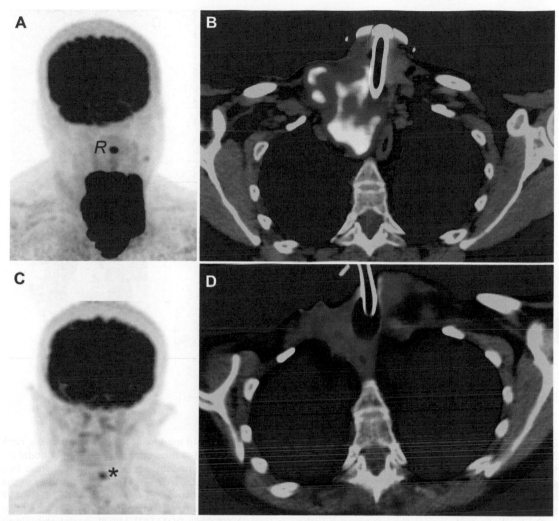

Fig. 7. A 65-year-old woman with anaplastic thyroid carcinoma had extrathyroidal extension and perineural invasion at surgery. Gross disease was left. Mutation testing showed BRAF V600E positivity. Postoperative FDG PET MIP in (*A*) and axial fused FDG PET/CT in (*B*) show residual right thyroid bed anaplastic thyroid carcinoma (SUV 41). A right lateral retropharyngeal nodal metastasis is also noted (*R*). Dabrafenib and trametinib therapy was started a week later. External beam radiation therapy to the right neck was completed. FDG PET MIP (*C*) and FDG PET/CT (*D*) obtained 19 months after (*A*) and (*B*) show complete metabolic response. Physiologic activity at the left cricoid cartilage is incidentally noted (*).

in 7 out of 14 scans.[40] Another study by Pryma and colleagues reported a sensitivity of 95.8% and a specificity of 95% for FDG PET/CT in HCTC (n = 44). They also demonstrated prognostic value of FDG PET/CT with a 6% increase in mortality for each unit increase in SUVmax.[41]

Anaplastic Thyroid Carcinoma

ATC is one of the most aggressive solid tumors with median survival time of about 6 to 8 months. It metastasizes frequently to lungs and bone with extensive local tissue invasion in greater than 70% of the patients.[42] These frequently dividing

tumor cells are unable to concentrate iodine or produce Tg but instead show high FDG uptake due to high glucose metabolism. ATA recommends FDG PET/CT in the evaluation of surgical resectability and localization of distant metastases, especially bone lesions.[43] In addition to its role in initial staging, PET is also a valuable tool in the follow-up of patients with ATC. FDG PET/CT has a higher sensitivity for detection of metastatic lesions than CT alone (99.6% vs 62% in identifying 265 individual lesions in 18 patients, P<.002) and resulted in treatment modification in 25% of cases.[44] FDG PET is also recommended 3 to 6 months after therapy in patients with no

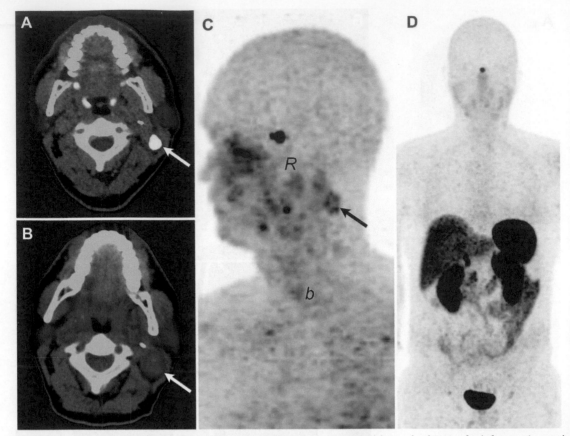

Fig. 8. Five years after diagnosis of medullary thyroid cancer, a 50-year-old man had FNA of a left superior neck node revealing metastasis. Calcitonin was 5.9. Axial fused FDG PET/CT in (*A*) showed left superior neck nodal activity, corresponding to site of FNA (*arrow*). The left lateral retropharyngeal node and the left thyroid bed showed similar levels of focal activity (not shown). (*B*) Axial fused Ga68-DOTATATE PET/CT shows activity in the left superior neck nodal metastasis (*arrow*) similar to adjacent parotid gland. (*C*) Ga68-DOTATATE PET/CT MIP shows mild activity in the left lateral retropharyngeal node (below *R*) and left thyroid bed (left of *b*), similar to the level of activity seen in the left superior neck node (*arrow*). (*D*) Ga68-DOTATATE MIP illustrates physiologic distribution of radiotracer in the pituitary gland, liver, spleen, urinary tract, and bowel.

disease or in persistent structural disease as a guide to therapy (**Fig. 7**). It may be useful in distinguishing ATC from DTC metastases because of the higher FDG uptake of ATC.[43] Poisson and colleagues showed that the volume (≥300 mL) and the intensity (SUVmax ≥18) of FDG uptake were significant negative prognostic factors for survival.[44]

Medullary Thyroid Carcinoma

MTCs generally display low avidity for FDG, therefore FDG PET/CT is not recommended for staging or for detection of distant metastases.[45] About half of patients (50%) with MTCs will have persistent or recurrent disease, despite primary surgical treatment (**Fig. 8**). If the postoperative serum calcitonin level exceeds 150 pg/mL, ATA 2015 guidelines recommend that these patients should be evaluated by imaging procedures, including neck US, chest CT, contrast-enhanced CT/MR imaging of the liver, bone scintigraphy, and MR imaging of the pelvis and axial skeleton.[45] FDG PET/CT has been found to be useful in patients with biochemical evidence of recurrence with detection rate (DR) of 50% and a lesion-based sensitivity of 96%.[46] Although FDG has high sensitivity for nodal metastases, it has lower sensitivity for lung and liver metastases.[47] In a meta-analysis of 24 studies comprising 538 patients with suspected recurrent MTC, DR of FDG PET/CT on a per patient–based analysis was 59% (95% CI: 54%–63%), and it increased to 75% when the calcitonin level was greater than 1000 ng/mL and decreased to 40% when it was less than 150 ng/mL[48]; this suggests that FDG PET/CT can be useful for assessing advanced disease with rapid progression

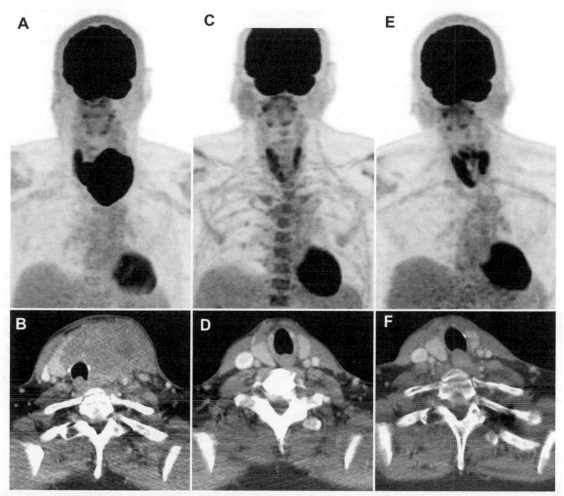

Fig. 9. A 63-year-old man had core biopsy of a thyroid mass, showing diffuse large B-cell lymphoma. (A) FDG PET MIP and (B) axial CT with contrast showed the left thyroid lymphoma with SUV 37 displacing the trachea to the right. Three months later after treatment, FDG PET MIP (C) showed decreased metabolic activity with SUV 3.8. Concurrent post contrast axial CT in (D) showed normal size of the thyroid gland in keeping with treatment response. Six months after FDG PET in (A), FDG PET MIP (E) showed moderate diffuse metabolic activity in the thyroid, SUV 9.6. Given the normal size of the thyroid gland in concurrent post contrast axial CT in (F), the increasing diffuse thyroid activity was likely due to treatment-related thyroiditis.

characterized by markedly elevated biochemical markers and shorter calcitonin doubling time.[49]

Gallium-68 (68 Ga) somatostatin analogue PET reflects expression of somatostatin receptors in MTC. Its use for feasibility of radionuclide therapy is being explored.[50,51] Although 68Ga-somatostatin analogue PET/CT is not recommended for staging, it can be useful in the settings of recurrent and metastatic disease. It is highly sensitive in detecting bone lesions (100%) and could be a substitute for a bone scan and MR imaging. In a retrospective study, a patient-based analysis showed more lesions on DOTATATE PET/CT (in 15/22 patients, 68.2% sensitivity) compared with FDG PET/CT (8/18, 44.4% sensitivity). DOTATATE PET/CT

seems to be an efficient imaging modality in patients with MTC with increased biochemical markers (calcitonin >1000 pg/mL) for localizing recurrent or metastatic disease.[52]

[18]F-fluorodihydroxyphenylalanine (^{18}F-DOPA) PET/CT has a higher sensitivity and is superior to FDG PET/CT and whole-body MR imaging in detecting and locating smaller unidentified lesions in patients with recurrent MTC with calcitonin greater than 150 ng/mL.[53] The superiority of F-DOPA uptake in MTC metastases comes from the fact that it is taken up by amino acid transporters and undergoes intracellular decarboxylation, which is a characteristic of cells of neuroendocrine origin. In a retrospective analysis

by Treglia and colleagues, F-DOPA detected more lesions in both patient- as well as lesion-based analyses.[54] In another study, F-DOPA PET detected significantly more lesions (75%, 56/75) compared with FDG PET (47%, 35/75) in 21 patients ($P = .009$).[55] FDG can be complementary to ^{18}F-DOPA PET/CT with DOPA having a higher sensitivity in detecting tumor load and FDG being more accurate in identifying progression and aggressive disease.[56]

Thyroid Lymphoma

Primary thyroid lymphoma is a rare entity, which typically develops in a setting of preexisting Hashimoto's thyroiditis.[57] It presents clinically as rapidly growing goiter and behaves as a high-grade malignant pathology. The diagnosis is made by US and FNA or core biopsy, with the most common pathology being diffuse large B-cell lymphoma.[58] To determine the local extent of disease, such as extrathyroidal spread, tracheal invasion, and lymph node involvement, CT and MR imaging are more useful than US. Because systemic disease is common in lymphomas, a CT of the chest, abdomen/pelvis, PET/CT, and bone marrow biopsy are required for staging.[59] FDG PET is an established study in the staging of lymphoma and has been proved to be superior to CT in detecting bone marrow infiltration and equivalent to bone marrow biopsy. Although FDG PET is positive in the primary lesion, it is also positive in autoimmune thyroiditis.[60] Nakadate and colleagues suggested the use of SUVmax (cut off = 14.1) to differentiate primary thyroid lymphoma from chronic thyroiditis on an FDG PET/CT scan. Primary thyroid lymphoma showed significantly higher FDG uptake (25.3 vs 7.4; $P<.001$) and lower CT density compared with those with chronic thyroiditis.[61] Basu and colleagues proved the clinical utility of FDG PET in initial staging and response assessment in thyroid lymphoma (Fig. 9). They also showed disease recurrence was detected earlier by FDG PET compared with CT.[62]

Other Radiopharmaceuticals

As discussed earlier, non-FDG PET radiotracers such as ^{18}F-DOPA and ^{68}Ga somatostatin analogues have been evaluated for specific types of thyroid cancers. Iodine-124 ([124]I) PET is another radiotracer that has greater spatial resolution than ^{131}I-WBS, and it can be used for detection of recurrent or residual DTC with considerably lower radiation exposure.[63] Iodine-124 PET is a sensitive tool to detect RAI avid DTC lesions,

with a pooled sensitivity of 94.2% (CI 91.3%–96.4%) in a recent meta-analysis.[64] In a review by Wu and colleagues including 6 studies using [124]I PET/CT, [124]I PET detected 120 lesions compared with 52 lesions on diagnostic ^{131}I scans in 72 patients. [124]I PET also detected 410 lesions compared with 390 lesions on posttherapy ^{131}I scans in 266 patients. TNM staging was revised in 15% to 21% of patients, and management was changed in 5% to 29% of patients.[65] Additional metastatic lesions detection by [124]I PET may have a significant clinical impact in the management of patients.

SUMMARY

The role of FDG PET/CT is evolving in the management of thyroid cancers. Incidental focal FDG uptake in thyroid carries a risk of malignancy, to be further evaluated in the context of any serious comorbidities. The most widely accepted role of FDG PET is in the evaluation of disease recurrence in patients with DTC when thyroglobulin levels are elevated along with a negative iodine scintigraphy. Furthermore, it can be used in initial staging of aggressive tumors such as HCTC, and ATC and has substantial future prospects in prognostication. FDG has also been shown to affect the management of high-risk progressive disease and can be extremely valuable in assessing response to systemic therapies. Because the role of ^{18}F-FDG is limited in MTC, other tracers such as ^{68}Ga-DOTATATE and ^{18}F-DOPA have been explored and can be considered in detecting recurrent or metastatic disease.

CLINICS CARE POINTS

- Immunotherapy can cause thyroiditis, which can be identified on FDG PET/CT obtained for response assessment.
- FDG PET/CT is not indicated for initial staging of DTC.
- FDG PET/CT is more likely to identify metastasis of thyroid cancer at higher serum levels of tumor markers.

DISCLOSURE

There are no relevant commercial or financial conflicts of interest or funding sources for any of the authors.

ACKNOWLEDGMENTS

The authors would like to thank Ms Kelly Kage for her kind assistance with the figures.

REFERENCES

1. Li M, Maso LD, Vaccarella S. Global trends in thyroid cancer incidence and the impact of overdiagnosis. Lancet Diabetes Endocrinol 2020;8(6):468–70.

2. Cancer of the Thyroid - Cancer Stat Facts. SEER. Available at: https://seer.cancer.gov/statfacts/html/thyro.html. Accessed November 12, 2020.

3. WHO classification. Available at: http://www.pathologyoutlines.com/topic/thyroidwho.html. Accessed November 12, 2020.

4. Fagin JA, Wells SA. Biologic and clinical perspectives on thyroid cancer. N Engl J Med 2016; 375(11):1054–67.

5. Ito Y, Miyauchi A, Kihara M, et al. Overall survival of papillary thyroid carcinoma patients: a single-institution long-term follow-up of 5897 patients. World J Surg 2018;42(3):615–22.

6. Randle RW, Balentine CJ, Leverson GE, et al. Trends in the presentation, treatment, and survival of patients with medullary thyroid cancer over the past 30 years. Surgery 2017;161(1):137–46.

7. Zhou X, Zheng Z, Chen C, et al. Clinical characteristics and prognostic factors of Hurthle cell carcinoma: a population based study. BMC Cancer 2020;20(1):407.

8. Survival Rates for Thyroid Cancer. Available at: https://www.cancer.org/cancer/thyroid-cancer/detection-diagnosis-staging/survival-rates.html. Accessed November 12, 2020.

9. Available at: thyroid.pdf https://www.nccn.org/professionals/physician_gls/pdf/thyroid.pdf. Accessed November 18, 2020.

10. Fletcher JW, Djulbegovic B, Soares HP, et al. Recommendations on the use of 18F-FDG PET in oncology. J Nucl Med 2008;49(3):480–508.

11. Haugen BR, Alexander EK, Bible KC, et al. 2015 American Thyroid Association Management Guidelines for Adult Patients with Thyroid Nodules and Differentiated Thyroid Cancer: The American Thyroid Association Guidelines Task Force on Thyroid Nodules and Differentiated Thyroid Cancer. Thyroid 2015;26(1):1–133.

12. Tessler FN, Middleton WD, Grant EG, et al. ACR Thyroid Imaging, Reporting and Data System (TI-RADS): White Paper of the ACR TI-RADS Committee. J Am Coll Radiol 2017;14(5):587–95.

13. Middleton WD, Teefey SA, Reading CC, et al. Multi-institutional Analysis of Thyroid Nodule Risk Stratification Using the American College of Radiology Thyroid Imaging Reporting and Data System. AJR Am J Roentgenol 2017;208(6):1331–41.

14. Choi JS, Kim J, Kwak JY, et al. Preoperative Staging of Papillary Thyroid Carcinoma: Comparison of Ultrasound Imaging and CT. Am J Roentgenol 2009; 193(3):871–8.

15. Ronga G, Filesi M, Montesano T, et al. Lung metastases from differentiated thyroid carcinoma. A 40 years' experience. Q J Nucl Med Mol Imaging 2004;48(1):12–9.

16. Treglia G, Giovanella L, Bertagna F, et al. Prevalence and risk of malignancy of thyroid incidentalomas detected by (18)f-fluorodeoxyglucose positron-emission tomography. Thyroid 2013;23(1):124–6.

17. Makis W, Ciarallo A, Probst S. Primary Thyroid Lymphoma: External Beam Radiation Therapy Induced Thyroiditis Mimics Residual Disease on Serial 18F-FDG PET/CT Imaging. Mol Imaging Radionucl Ther 2018;27(1):41–7.

18. Wang X, Wang J, Yang X, et al. Pembrolizumab Exacerbates Thyroid Diseases Shown on FDG PET/CT. Clin Nucl Med 2020;45(12):1010–2.

19. Eshghi N, Garland LL, Nia E, et al. 18F-FDG PET/CT Can Predict Development of Thyroiditis Due to Immunotherapy for Lung Cancer. J Nucl Med Technol 2018;46(3):260–4.

20. Soelberg KK, Bonnema SJ, Brix TH, et al. Risk of Malignancy in Thyroid Incidentalomas Detected by 18F-Fluorodeoxyglucose Positron Emission Tomography: A Systematic Review. Thyroid 2012;22(9): 918–25.

21. Hoang JK, Langer JE, Middleton WD, et al. Managing incidental thyroid nodules detected on imaging: white paper of the ACR Incidental Thyroid Findings Committee. J Am Coll Radiol 2015; 12(2):143–50.

22. Bertagna F, Treglia G, Piccardo A, et al. Diagnostic and clinical significance of F-18-FDG-PET/CT thyroid incidentalomas. J Clin Endocrinol Metab 2012; 97(11):3866–75.

23. Castellana M, Trimboli P, Piccardo A, et al. Performance of 18F-FDG PET/CT in Selecting Thyroid Nodules with Indeterminate Fine-Needle Aspiration Cytology for Surgery. A Systematic Review and a Meta-Analysis. J Clin Med 2019;8(9). https://doi.org/10.3390/jcm8091333.

24. Piccardo A, Puntoni M, Dezzana M, et al. Indeterminate thyroid nodules. The role of 18F-FDG PET/CT in the "era" of ultrasonography risk stratification systems and new thyroid cytology classifications. Endocrine 2020;69(3):553–61.

25. Vriens D, Adang EMM, Netea-Maier RT, et al. Cost-effectiveness of FDG-PET/CT for cytologically indeterminate thyroid nodules: a decision analytic approach. J Clin Endocrinol Metab 2014;99(9): 3263–74.

26. Deandreis D, Al Ghuzlan A, Auperin A, et al. Is 18F-Fluorodeoxyglucose–PET/CT Useful for the Presurgical Characterization of Thyroid Nodules with

Indeterminate Fine Needle Aspiration Cytology? Thyroid 2012;22(2):165–72.

27. Qichang W, Lin B, Gege Z, et al. Diagnostic performance of 18F-FDG-PET/CT in DTC patients with thyroglobulin elevation and negative iodine scintigraphy: a meta-analysis. Eur J Endocrinol 2019; 181(2):93–102.

28. Lebouleux S, Schroeder PR, Schlumberger M, et al. The role of PET in follow-up of patients treated for differentiated epithelial thyroid cancers. Nat Clin Pract Endocrinol Metab 2007;3(2):112–21.

29. Schütz F, Lautenschläger C, Lorenz K, et al. Positron Emission Tomography (PET) and PET/CT in Thyroid Cancer: A Systematic Review and Meta-Analysis. Eur Thyroid J 2018;7(1):13–20.

30. Kim D-H, Kim S-J. Diagnostic role of F-18 FDG PET/CT for preoperative lymph node staging in thyroid cancer patients; A systematic review and metaanalysis. Clin Imaging 2020;65:100–7.

31. Kim S-J, Lee S-W, Pak K, et al. Diagnostic performance of PET in thyroid cancer with elevated anti-Tg Ab. Endocr Relat Cancer 2018;25(6):643–52.

32. Fugazzola L, Elisei R, Fuhrer D, et al. 2019 European Thyroid Association Guidelines for the Treatment and Follow-Up of Advanced Radioiodine-Refractory Thyroid Cancer. Eur Thyroid J 2019; 8(5):227–45.

33. Piccardo A, Trimboli P, Foppiani L, et al. PET/CT in thyroid nodule and differentiated thyroid cancer patients. The evidence-based state of the art. Rev Endocr Metab Disord 2019;20(1):47–64.

34. Vural GU, Akkas BE, Ercakmak N, et al. Prognostic significance of FDG PET/CT on the follow-up of patients of differentiated thyroid carcinoma with negative 131I whole-body scan and elevated thyroglobulin levels: correlation with clinical and histopathologic characteristics and long-term follow-up data. Clin Nucl Med 2012;37(10):953–9.

35. Salvatore B, Klain M, Nicolai E, et al. Prognostic role of FDG PET/CT in patients with differentiated thyroid cancer treated with 131-iodine empiric therapy. Medicine (Baltimore) 2017;96(42).

36. Deandreis D, Al Ghuzlan A, Lebouleux S, et al. Do histological, immunohistochemical, and metabolic (radioiodine and fluorodeoxyglucose uptakes) patterns of metastatic thyroid cancer correlate with patient outcome? Endocr Relat Cancer 2011;18(1): 159–69.

37. Larg MI, Barbus E, Gabora K, et al. 18F-FDG PET/CT in differentiated thyroid carcinoma. Acta Endocrinol (Buchar) 2019;15(2):203–8.

38. Pathak KA, Klonisch T, Nason RW, et al. FDG-PET characteristics of Hürthle cell and follicular adenomas. Ann Nucl Med 2016;30(7):506–9.

39. Treglia G, Annunziata S, Muoio B, et al. The role of fluorine-18-fluorodeoxyglucose positron emission tomography in aggressive histological subtypes of

thyroid cancer: an overview. Int J Endocrinol 2013. https://doi.org/10.1155/2013/856189.

40. Lowe VJ, Mullan BP, Hay ID, et al. 18F-FDG PET of Patients with Hürthle Cell Carcinoma. J Nucl Med 2003;44(9):1402–6.

41. Pryma DA, Schöder H, Gönen M, et al. Diagnostic Accuracy and Prognostic Value of 18F-FDG PET in Hürthle Cell Thyroid Cancer Patients. J Nucl Med 2006;47(8):1260–6.

42. Chiacchio S, Lorenzoni A, Boni G, et al. Anaplastic thyroid cancer: prevalence, diagnosis and treatment. Minerva Endocrinol 2008;33(4):341–57.

43. Smallridge RC, Ain KB, Asa SL, et al. American Thyroid Association guidelines for management of patients with anaplastic thyroid cancer. Thyroid 2012; 22(11):1104–39.

44. Poisson T, Deandreis D, Lebouleux S, et al. 18F-fluorodeoxyglucose positron emission tomography and computed tomography in anaplastic thyroid cancer. Eur J Nucl Med Mol Imaging 2010;37(12):2277–85.

45. Wells SA, Asa SL, Dralle H, et al. Revised American Thyroid Association Guidelines for the Management of Medullary Thyroid Carcinoma. Thyroid 2015; 25(6):567–610.

46. de Groot JWB, Links TP, Jager PL, et al. Impact of 18F-fluoro-2-deoxy-D-glucose positron emission tomography (FDG-PET) in patients with biochemical evidence of recurrent or residual medullary thyroid cancer. Ann Surg Oncol 2004;11(8):786–94.

47. Ganeshan D, Paulson E, Duran C, et al. Current Update on Medullary Thyroid Carcinoma. Am J Roentgenol 2013;201(6):W867–76.

48. Treglia G, Villani MF, Giordano A, et al. Detection rate of recurrent medullary thyroid carcinoma using fluorine-18 fluorodeoxyglucose positron emission tomography: a meta-analysis. Endocrine 2012;42(3): 535–45.

49. Yang JH, Camacho CP, Lindsey SC, et al. THE COMBINED USE OF CALCITONIN DOUBLING TIME AND 18F-FDG PET/CT IMPROVES PROGNOSTIC VALUES IN MEDULLARY THYROID CARCINOMA: THE CLINICAL UTILITY OF 18F-FDG PET/CT. Endocr Pract 2017;23(8):942–8.

50. Virgolini I, Gabriel M, Kroiss A, et al. Current knowledge on the sensitivity of the (68)Ga-somatostatin receptor positron emission tomography and the SUVmax reference range for management of pancreatic neuroendocrine tumours. Eur J Nucl Med Mol Imaging 2016;43(11):2072–83.

51. Parghane RV, Naik C, Talole S, et al. Clinical utility of 177Lu-DOTATATE PRRT in somatostatin receptor-positive metastatic medullary carcinoma of thyroid patients with assessment of efficacy, survival analysis, prognostic variables, and toxicity. Head Neck 2020;42(3):401–16.

52. Ozkan ZG, Kuyumcu S, Uzum AK, et al. Comparison of 68Ga-DOTATATE PET-CT, 18F-FDG PET-CT and

99mTc-(V)DMSA scintigraphy in the detection of recurrent or metastatic medullary thyroid carcinoma. Nucl Med Commun 2015;36(3):242–50.

53. Romero-Lluch AR, Cuenca-Cuenca JI, Guerrero-Vázquez R, et al. Diagnostic utility of PET/CT with 18F-DOPA and 18F-FDG in persistent or recurrent medullary thyroid carcinoma: the importance of calcitonin and carcinoembryonic antigen cutoff. Eur J Nucl Med Mol Imaging 2017;44(12):2004–13.

54. Treglia G, Castaldi P, Villani MF, et al. Comparison of 18F-DOPA, 18F-FDG and 68Ga-somatostatin analogue PET/CT in patients with recurrent medullary thyroid carcinoma. Eur J Nucl Med Mol Imaging 2012;39(4):569–80.

55. Verbeek HHG, Plukker JTM, Koopmans KP, et al. Clinical Relevance of 18F-FDG PET and 18F-DOPA PET in Recurrent Medullary Thyroid Carcinoma. J Nucl Med 2012;53(12):1863–71.

56. Kauhanen S, Schalin-Jäntti C, Seppänen M, et al. Complementary roles of 18F-DOPA PET/CT and 18F-FDG PET/CT in medullary thyroid cancer. J Nucl Med 2011;52(12):1855–63.

57. Walsh S, Lowery AJ, Evoy D, et al. Thyroid lymphoma: recent advances in diagnosis and optimal management strategies. Oncologist 2013;18(9):994–1003.

58. Kesireddy M, Lasrado S. Thyroid Lymphoma. In: StatPearls [Internet]. Treasure Island (FL): StatPearls Publishing; 2020. Available at: http://www.ncbi.nlm.nih.gov/books/NBK544282/.

59. Spielman DB, Badhey A, Kadakia S, et al. Rare thyroid malignancies: an overview for the oncologist. Clin Oncol 2017;29(5):298–306.

60. Małkowski B, Serafin Z, Glonek R, et al. The Role of 18F-FDG PET/CT in the Management of the Autoimmune Thyroid Diseases. Front Endocrinol 2019;10. https://doi.org/10.3389/fendo.2019.00208.

61. Nakadate M, Yoshida K, Ishii A, et al. Is 18F-FDG PET/CT useful for distinguishing between primary thyroid lymphoma and chronic thyroiditis? Clin Nucl Med 2013;38(9):709–14.

62. Basu S, Li G, Bural G, et al. Fluorodeoxyglucose positron emission tomography (FDG-PET) and PET/computed tomography imaging characteristics of thyroid lymphoma and their potential clinical utility. Acta Radiol Stockh Swed 2009;50(2):201–4.

63. Marcus C, Whitworth PW, Surasi DS, et al. PET/CT in the management of thyroid cancers. Am J Roentgenol 2014;202(6):1316–29.

64. Santhanam P, Taieb D, Solnes L, et al. Utility of I-124 PET/CT in identifying radioiodine avid lesions in differentiated thyroid cancer: a systematic review and meta-analysis. Clin Endocrinol (Oxf) 2017; 86(5):645–51.

65. Wu D, Ylli D, Heimlich SL, et al. 124I Positron Emission Tomography/Computed Tomography Versus Conventional Radioiodine Imaging in Differentiated Thyroid Cancer: A Review. Thyroid 2019;29(11):1523–35.

Management of Anaplastic and Recurrent Differentiated Thyroid Cancer
Indications for Surgical Resection, Molecular Testing, and Systemic Therapy

Maria E. Cabanillas, MD[a],*, Salmaan Ahmed, MD[b],
Jennifer Rui Wang, MD, ScM[c]

KEYWORDS

- Kinase inhibitor • BRAF • MEK • RET • NTRK

KEY POINTS

- Major advancements in the treatment of advanced thyroid cancer have emerged in large part because of a better understanding of the genetic drivers.
- Anaplastic thyroid cancer, previously thought to be uniformly fatal, is now treatable, particularly if the tumor harbors a *BRAF* mutation and can be targeted with BRAF inhibitors. Other targeted agents are promising for non–*BRAF*-mutated anaplastic thyroid cancer.
- There are 5 US Food and Drug Administration approved drugs for differentiated thyroid cancer, including pathway inhibitors (antiangiogenic drugs) and selective inhibitors of NTRK and RET.

INTRODUCTION

Thyroid carcinoma comprises several different types of cancers, which include those derived from the follicular epithelial thyroid cells (differentiated thyroid cancer [DTC] and anaplastic thyroid cancer [ATC]), the C cells of the thyroid (medullary thyroid cancer), and the lymphocytes of the thyroid gland (thyroid lymphomas). This article focuses on the tumors derived from the follicular epithelial cells of the thyroid, which are cells that normally trap iodine and produce thyroid hormone.

There are 3 types of DTC tumors: papillary thyroid cancer (PTC; 85% of DTCs), follicular thyroid cancer (FTC; 10% of DTCs), and Hürthle cell thyroid cancer (HTC; 5% of DTCs). These tumors may dedifferentiate, losing some (poorly differentiated) or all (ATC) of the typical pathologic characteristics that define the DTCs, become necrotic,

lose the ability to take up radioactive iodine (RAI), and behave more aggressively. Hürthle cell thyroid cancers are particularly difficult to manage because they are usually RAI refractory. Poorly differentiated thyroid carcinoma is categorized as a DTC but these are derived from PTCs, FTCs, and HTCs.

ATC is an undifferentiated thyroid cancer, meaning it has none of the pathologic features that characterize the DTC tumors, but they are thought to derive from these tumors as the end stage of dedifferentiation. It is likely that acquisition of new mutations is what results in ATC. These tumors are the most aggressive and rare form of thyroid cancer, but are treated, and should be thought of, as several subtypes of ATC, based on the tumor from which they are derived. This condition is often identified either because there is a DTC subtype coexisting with the ATC or

[a] Departments of Endocrine Neoplasia and Hormonal Disorders, The University of Texas MD Anderson Cancer Center, 1515 Holcombe Boulevard, Unit 1461, Houston, TX 77030, USA; [b] Diagnostic Imaging, The University of Texas MD Anderson Cancer Center, 1515 Holcombe Boulevard, Houston, TX 77030, USA; [c] Head and Neck Surgery, The University of Texas MD Anderson Cancer Center, 1515 Holcombe Boulevard, Houston, TX 77030, USA
* Corresponding author.
E-mail address: mcabani@mdanderson.org

Neuroimag Clin N Am 31 (2021) 359–366
https://doi.org/10.1016/j.nic.2021.04.005
1052-5149/21/© 2021 Elsevier Inc. All rights reserved.

from the driver mutations (discussed next). Patients may also have a history of DTC that transformed to ATC. The resulting ATC tumors retain the driver mutation from the parent DTC from which it was derived.

MOLECULAR PROFILE

Several next-generation sequencing (NGS) studies have been performed for DTC, the largest being The Cancer Genome Atlas (TCGA) project, where 507 patients with PTC were profiled.[1] In general, PTC is characterized by a low frequency of somatic mutations. BRAF is the most frequently mutated gene, found in approximately 60% of tumors, where the almost all involve a missense mutation where valine is substituted by glutamic acid at amino acid 600 (BRAFV600E). Mutations in other genes occur at low frequencies (<10%), including mutations in the RAS family of genes (NRAS, HRAS, KRAS), which are mutually exclusive with one another and BRAF. TERT promoter mutations were identified in 9% of tumors, which showed an association with high-risk features. Moreover, chromosomal rearrangements and translocations were identified in 15%, with RET fusions being most common.[1] Similar to PTC, FTC is characterized by frequent alterations in the mitogen-activated protein kinase (MAPK) pathway. However, RAS mutations and PAX8/PPARγ fusions occur more commonly in FTC.[2]

Compared with DTC, ATC is characterized by a higher mutation burden with increased rates of alterations in tumors suppressors (TP53), PI3K/AKT pathway genes, and the TERT promoter. Although TP53 mutations are rare in PTC (<5%), it can be identified in up to 70% of ATC tumors, thereby serving as a molecular hallmark of ATC. Similarly, TERT promoter mutations were identified in approximately 40% of ATC tumors. The BRAFV600E mutation is found in 25% to 40% of tumors, which are generally mutually exclusive with mutations in RAS genes (NRAS, KRAS, HRAS) pretreatment.[3–7] The third molecular subgroup is made up of the remaining tumors without BRAFV600E and RAS mutations where putative driver mutations are varied and incompletely described.[3]

MANAGEMENT

Recurrent or Metastatic Differentiated Thyroid Cancer

Observation, also called the watch-and-wait approach, is sometimes warranted for DTC. This decision depends on whether the location of the recurrent or metastatic disease will result in imminent morbidity if left in place. The watch-and-wait approach is favored for distant metastatic disease because (1) most patients with DTC have indolent disease; (2) distant metastatic disease is usually incurable, except for some with RAI-sensitive disease, and systemic therapy (such as with kinase inhibitors) does not lead to complete responses in most cases; (3) systemic therapy potentially has many adverse effects that can diminish the quality of life of patients, and these drugs are used as continuous therapy until no longer effective or the patients experience an intolerable adverse event that cannot be treated effectively. It should be stressed that TSH-suppressive therapy should always accompany any form of therapy, especially watch and wait.

Localized therapies, such as radiation and embolization, are also considered for metastatic DTC. Although external beam radiation to gross DTC in the neck is discouraged, focused beam radiation, such as stereotactic beam radiation therapy, may be used for management of bone, brain, and metastases to other organs. In the spine and brain, stereotactic radiation is used to avoid a catastrophic outcome such as paralysis. However, beyond the central nervous system, stereotactic radiation is also used to treat, but is not limited to, axial bone, lung, liver, and even abdominal nodal metastases. Embolization of large tumors such as bone or liver has also been used to manage DTC. Stereotactic radiation, preferred for smaller burden of disease, and embolization, preferred for larger tumors, may delay systemic therapy. These methods may also be used in patients with high risk of local complications such as fracture or postobstructive pneumonia.

For locally recurrent DTC, watch and wait may also be used for some of the same reasons. If feasible, surgery may result in morbidity (ie, vocal cord paralysis, hypoparathyroidism, shoulder dysfunction, fibrosis, dysphagia) and diminished quality of life of the patients. Particularly in patients with distant metastases, surgery may not be curative, thus weighing the risk/benefit ratio and discussing this with the patient is prudent. Alcohol ablation therapy may be considered in appropriate patients.

The most common site of persistent or recurrent DTC is in the cervical lymph nodes, usually identified by neck ultrasonography. Disease can involve the central neck and/or lateral neck. Recurrence and/or persistent disease involving the central compartment is more common than lateral neck disease. Progressive, uncontrolled central neck disease can pose significant risks to surrounding structures, including risks to recurrent laryngeal nerves, trachea, and/or esophagus. Although redo surgery is associated with increased risks caused by prior scarring and issues such as preexisting vocal cord paralysis, it has been shown that, in experienced hands, comprehensive central compartment dissection is a reproducible and safe procedure in patients with recurrent or persistence DTC.[8] In patients with small-volume disease (<1 cm), particularly in patients with preexisting unilateral vocal cord paralysis, the risks and timing of surgery must be weighed against potential benefits. Intraoperative recurrent laryngeal nerve monitoring is an important adjunct in redo central compartment surgery. In patients with recurrent or persistent lateral neck disease, comprehensive dissection to remove lymph nodes from levels II to V is advocated as opposed to a limited cherry-picking approach to address isolated lymph node disease. Persistent thyroglobulinemia in the setting of a normal neck ultrasonography scan should prompt cross-sectional imaging with contrast of the neck and chest in order to identify disease in the retropharyngeal nodes and below the clavicles in the mediastinum, hilum, and lungs. Although patients can develop recurrence in the lateral neck outside of levels II to V (ie, retropharyngeal lymph nodes), these are rare.[9] In patients with locally advanced disease (ie, significant extra-thyroidal extension), more extensive surgical procedures may be required to address recurrent disease, such as tracheal resection, mediastinal dissection, and reconstruction. These procedures should be performed at tertiary care centers with surgical expertise in the management of advanced thyroid cancers.

Systemic therapy for DTC can be divided into the predominantly antiangiogenic, multikinase-inhibitor drugs and drugs that target a specific mutation or fusion in the tumor. The two US Food and Drug Administration (FDA)–approved antiangiogenic drugs are the multikinase inhibitors sorafenib and lenvatinib. Sorafenib targets vascular endothelial growth factor (VEGF) 1 to 3, platelet-derived growth factor (PDGF), fibroblast growth factor (FGF), and KIT and RET receptors. The drug is approved for I-131–refractory DTC, renal cell carcinoma, and hepatocellular carcinoma. The drug was approved for DTC based on the DECISION trial.[10] This trial was a double-blinded, placebo-controlled study that included 417 patients with I-131–refractory DTC, 207 of whom were randomized to sorafenib, and 209 to placebo. All patients in this trial were kinase inhibitor naive. The median progression-free survival was 10.8 months with sorafenib versus 5.8 months in the placebo arm (hazard ratio [HR], 0.59; 95% confidence interval [CI], 0.45–0.76; P<.0001). Crossover was

permitted, limiting the analysis of overall survival, but the median did not differ between the 2 arms.

Lenvatinib is also a VEGF 1 to 3 receptor inhibitor. It also targets FGF1 to 4, PDGF, and KIT and RET receptors. It is a more potent antiangiogenic drug than sorafenib, and therefore some adverse events may be more severe. This drug is FDA approved as a single agent for I-131–refractory DTC and hepatocellular carcinoma. It is also approved for renal cell carcinoma in combination with everolimus. Lenvatinib was approved based on the SELECT trial, a double-blinded, placebo-controlled, randomized trial that included 261 patients in the lenvatinib arm and 131 in the placebo arm.[11] Patients were allowed 1 previous VEGF kinase inhibitor. The median progression-free survival was 18.3 months in the lenvatinib arm and 3.6 months in the placebo arm (HR, 0.21; 99% CI, 0.14–0.31; P<.001). Crossover was also permitted in this study and there was no statistically significant median overall survival benefit. However, in patients more than 65 years of age, there was a survival advantage (not reached) versus those randomized to placebo (18.4 months).

Relative contraindications for antiangiogenic therapy may preclude the use of these drugs in some patients[12] and are listed in Box 1. These contraindications were established because of the risk of hypertension, which may lead to cardiac dysfunction, poor wound healing, risks of bowel perforation, tracheoesophageal fistula,[13] and carotid blow-out.[14,15] Radiologists should be aware

---

Box 1
Relative contraindications to antiangiogenic drugs

Relative contraindications to potent antiangiogenic agents

Cardiac:

   Poor cardiac function or recent myocardial infarction

   Uncontrolled hypertension

Gastrointestinal:

   Previous history of, or active, colitis

   Previous history of diverticulitis

   Previous history of intestinal perforation

   Recent bowel surgery

Large, unhealed wounds

Tumor invading trachea, esophagus, or great vessels

Hemoptysis or use of anticoagulants

of these risks, because their input in multidisciplinary tumor boards is often sought. Other more targeted agents or lower starting doses of the drug may be considered if any of these contraindications exist.

Selective BRAF inhibitors are the most commonly used off-label alternative to the antiangiogenic drugs. These inhibitors are not FDA approved but have been investigated in DTC. There are 3 selective BRAF inhibitors that are commercially approved: vemurafenib, dabrafenib, and encorafenib. The first 2 have been studied in DTC. Vemurafenib is a selective BRAF inhibitor, FDA approved for *BRAF*-mutated melanoma, which was studied in a phase 2, nonrandomized trial in *BRAF*-mutated PTC.[16] Patients were stratified into 2 groups: treatment naive and previous VEGF receptor (VEGFR) inhibitor treatment. The primary end point was overall response in the treatment-naive patients. In this group, the partial response rate was 38.5% and the median progression-free survival was 18.2 months (95% CI, 15.5–29.3 months). As expected, the previously treated group had a lower response rate (27.3%) and shorter progression-free survival (8.9 months, 95% [CI, 5.5 months to not estimable]). Although the overall survival was not reached in the treatment-naive group, the overall survival was 14.4 months (95% CI, 8.2–29.5 months) in the patients previously treated with VEGFR inhibitor.

Dabrafenib is also a selective BRAF inhibitor, FDA approved for BRAF-mutated melanoma, ATC, and lung cancer. The drug has been studied in *BRAF*-mutated PTC in 2 clinical trials.[17,18] The second clinical trial was the larger of the 2 studies. This trial was randomized to 2 arms: dabrafenib alone and dabrafenib plus trametinib (a selective MEK inhibitor). Patients in the dabrafenib alone arm were allowed to cross over to the dual-therapy arm. In the single-agent arm, 10 out of 26 (38%) patients had a partial response to therapy, whereas, in the dual arm, 9 out of 27 (33%) had a partial response. The median progression-free survival was 11.4 months in the single-agent arm and 15.1 months in the dual-treatment arm.

Dabrafenib has also been reported to restore RAI uptake in tumors,[19] a treatment referred to as redifferentiation or resensitization. This trial enrolled 10 patients with *BRAF*-mutated, RAI-refractory PTC. Patients received dabrafenib for 25 days before undergoing diagnostic whole-body scan. Those who took up RAI were treated for another 17 days before receiving 150 mCi of I-131. Dabrafenib was then discontinued. Six of the 10 patients qualified to receive I-131 treatment, of whom 2 (33%) had a partial response after 3 months.

Selumetinib is a MEK inhibitor that is FDA approved for neurofibromatosis type 1 with symptomatic, inoperable plexiform neurofibromas. The strategy of redifferentiation has also been reported with this drug.[20] In this small proof-of-concept study, 20 patients with RAI-refractory DTC were treated for 4 weeks with selumetinib. Eight of these patients reached the necessary threshold for RAI therapy by dosimetry and received RAI. Selumetinib was then discontinued. Of these 8 patients, 5 had a partial response to RAI. Surprisingly, 4 of these patients with partial responses to RAI had NRAS mutations and only 1 had BRAFV600E mutation. None of the patients with RET/PTC fusions had RAI uptake. Although it is not known whether other selective inhibitors that affect signaling along the MAPK pathway will have the same effect on restoring RAI uptake, there has been 1 case report of this with the selective NTRK inhibitor larotrectinib.[21]

Fusion events such as *NTRK*, *RET*, and *ALK* fusions are rare drivers in DTC and ATC. There are several selective inhibitors that are approved for thyroid cancer. Larotrectinib and entrectinib are selective NTRK inhibitors that are FDA approved for any solid tumor with *NTRK* fusion, and seem to be highly effective in DTC. Of the 2 drugs, larotrectinib has reported the most data in thyroid cancer.[22,23] Data from an adult phase 1 trial and from an adult/adolescent phase 2 basket trial were combined. A total of 28 patients with *NTRK* fusion thyroid cancer were reported at ESMO (European Society for Medical Oncology) 2020.[23] There were 21 patients with DTC and 7 patients with ATC. The DTC group had a very high response rate of 90%, including 2 complete responses. The median progression-free survival was not reached in this group but, at 18 months, 86% were free of progression. The median overall survival was not reached in the DTC group.

Pralsetinib and selpercatinib are selective *RET* inhibitors. Both drugs are FDA approved for *RET*-altered thyroid and lung cancer. A phase 1/2 trial enrolled 19 patients with nonmedullary thyroid cancer with *RET* fusion: 13 with PTC, 3 with poorly differentiated thyroid cancer (PDTC), 1 Hürthle cell, and 2 with ATC.[24] Independent (centrally) reviewed response rate was 79%, including 1 complete response. At 1 year, 64% of the patients were progression free. In the pralsetinib clinical trial, 11 evaluable patients with *RET* fusion thyroid cancer were reported at ASCO (American Society of Clinical Oncology) 2020.[25] The overall response rate in this group was 91%, but it should be noted that there were no patients with ATC included.

Anaplastic Thyroid Cancer

As mentioned previously, ATC should not be thought of as one disease, but in relation to the DTC tumor from which it is derived, which may be obvious in the tumor specimen if there is a coexisting DTC or from the past medical history of the patient if the ATC is transformed from DTC. If the tumor harbors a BRAF mutation, it is PTC derived, and the prognosis is the most favorable of all types of ATC, because these patients are highly treatable. Thus, the approach to ATC should always begin with determination of the BRAF status. However, NGS testing is slow and waiting for this test to give results may lead to patients' demise before they can receive any treatment. Alternatively, BRAF testing by immunohistochemistry (IHC) is a rapid test that has been shown to be accurate for determining the BRAF status. This test should be performed on all newly diagnosed patients with ATC but NGS should also be sent in parallel, because approximately 60% of patients do not have a BRAF mutation. Molecular testing by NGS and BRAF by IHC is not always feasible and therefore a more rapid test is the liquid biopsy (circulating free DNA) test.

Treatment of ATC depends on the stage and the driver mutation or fusion. Stage IVA disease is localized to the thyroid gland and should be surgically resected then treated with external beam radiation to the neck, preferably with concurrent radiosensitizing chemotherapy. Stage IVB disease has gone beyond the capsule of the thyroid gland but has not metastasized outside of the neck. Upfront surgery should be considered; however, few stage IVB patients are considered to be meaningfully resectable. Most patients with T4b disease present with advanced disease that requires radical resection, such as total laryngectomy and/or esophagectomy. Given increased morbidity associated with radical resection, upfront surgery is avoided in most cases. In these patients, neoadjuvant treatment with a BRAF/MEK inhibitor should be considered for those with a BRAF mutation (discussed further later).

There are FDA-approved drugs for BRAF-mutated, RET-fusion, and NTRK-fusion ATC, but limited data exist for the last two. In 2018, the FDA approved dabrafenib plus trametinib for BRAFV600E-mutated ATC. This approval was based on a prospective, phase 2 clinical trial.[26] At the time of this publication, there were 16 evaluable patients. The overall response rate was 69% (with 1 complete response). The median overall survival had not been reached. An updated report presented at ESMO reported data on 28 patients enrolled on this trial.[27] The median progression-free and overall survival were 60 and 86 weeks, respectively.

Neoadjuvant treatment with BRAF/MEK inhibitors in patients with BRAFV600E-mutated ATC can significantly reduce the burden of disease and enable surgical resection, as shown in Figs. 1 and 2. The authors have shown in our initial experience that this approach is feasible in patients with ATC with advanced IVB disease and in selected patients whose limited distant disease responds favorably to neoadjuvant treatment.[28] In the use of this treatment approach, rapid diagnosis, ascertainment of BRAF mutation status, and treatment initiation are essential to avoid tracheostomy and local complications. Significant reduction in disease burden can be observed within days of treatment initiation, which may improve airway and swallowing symptoms. Restaging evaluation to determine surgical candidacy can be performed after 1 to 2 months of BRAF/MEK treatment. Before surgery, restaging with contrast-enhanced computed tomography (CT) neck is essential to determine resectability. In addition, PET/CT and magnetic resonance imaging brain should also be obtained to assess status of distant disease before surgery. In cases with known distant metastases, surgical resection of the primary and neck disease can be considered if distant disease has responded to neoadjuvant treatment and/or remains at low volume. Because of the antiangiogenic properties associated with MEK inhibitors, which can impair postsurgical sound healing, MEK inhibitor is held 5 to 7 days before surgery. BRAF inhibitor is held the day before or on the day of surgery. Both drugs are restarted as soon as the surgical wound has healed, typically within 1 to 2 weeks from surgery. At present, the addition of immunotherapy to BRAF/MEK is being evaluated in a neoadjuvant setting in a clinical trial.

The larotrectinib trial, a selective NTRK inhibitor, detailed earlier, enrolled 7 patients with ATC with NTRK fusion.[23] In the ATC cohort, 2 patients experienced a partial response (29%), whereas 1 patient had stable disease and 3 had progression (43%) as their best responses. The median overall survival in this group was 14.1 months. Because of the small numbers and lack of information regarding durability of response, it is unclear whether this will be a reasonable strategy for patients with ATC. No data have been reported in ATC with entrectinib. In the selpercatinib trial, a selective RET inhibitor, only 2 patients with ATC were reported. One of the 2 patients enrolled in the trial had a partial response to therapy, which was sustained for 18 months, with the response ongoing at the time of publication.

Patients who do not have a BRAF mutation or RET or NTRK fusion are complicated patients to

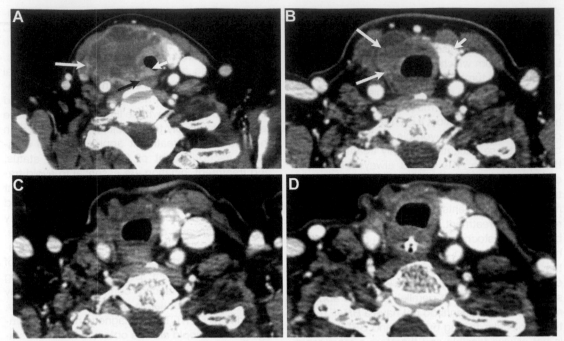

Fig. 1. A 77-year-old woman with right thyroid mass biopsy showing ATC. (*A*) Axial contrast-enhanced computed tomography (CECT) shows a large, heterogenous, partially necrotic, solid mass involving the right thyroid lobe and isthmus. There is direct invasion of the trachea (*small white arrow*) and esophagus (*black arrow*), and tumor infiltrates the right tracheoesophageal groove. Midline structures are displaced to the left. There is direct extension of tumor to the lateral compartment (*long white arrow*). Left lobe of the thyroid has a normal appearance. (*B*) Axial CECT obtained 4 months following initiation of dabrafenib and trametinib shows near resolution of the right lobe tumor. Trachea and esophageal involvement have resolved and small-volume residual soft tissue in the right central compartment is nonenhancing (*long arrows*). Normal left thyroid lobe (*short arrow*). (*C*) Right thyroid lobectomy and right central and lateral neck dissection were performed following 10 months of systemic therapy. Postoperative axial CECT shows no residual enhancement or soft tissue abnormality in the right central compartment. Pathology shows predominantly treatment-related change with less than 5% viable ATC. Three cervical lymph nodes showed DTC. (*D*) CECT obtained 11 months after surgery and 23 months after initial diagnosis of ATC is without evidence for large-volume recurrence in the central or lateral compartments. Residual left thyroid lobe remains normal.

manage. These patients should be referred for clinical trial, because it is not clear whether there are effective therapies. The only single-agent immunotherapy trial was published in 2020. This study, with and anti–programmed death-ligand 1 (PD-L1) inhibitor, spartalizumab,[29] showed an overall response rate of 19%. Median overall survival was 5.9 months and 40% of patients were alive at 1 year. When specimens were analyzed by PD-L1 expression, those with less than 1% expression did not respond to therapy, whereas those with more than 1% to 49% had a response rate of 20% and those with 50% or more had a response rate of 29%. Overall survival also correlated with PD-L1 expression. Specimens with less than 1% PD-L1 expression had a median overall survival of 1.6 months (95% CI, 1.0–19.6), whereas those with any PD-L1 expression had a median overall survival that was not reached. Seven

patients with *BRAF*V600E mutations were enrolled on this trial. Of these, only 1 patient had a partial response (14%), thus, the authors do not recommend single-agent immunotherapy for patients with *BRAF*V600E mutation because the response rates with BRAF/MEK inhibitors are far better.

Combination immunotherapy and combination targeted therapy and immunotherapy have also been investigated in ATC. In a combination nivolumab plus ipilimumab trial, 10 patients with ATC were enrolled.[30] Of 8 evaluable patients, 3 had a partial response. The median overall response in this group was 4.29 months (95% CI, 1.22 to not reached). PD-L1 and *BRAF* mutation status was not reported. Another trial with combination cobimetinib plus atezolizumab for patients with *RAS* or *NF-1*–mutated ATC showed a partial response rate of 17% with a median overall survival of 18.23 months (95% CI, 4.47–NE).[31]

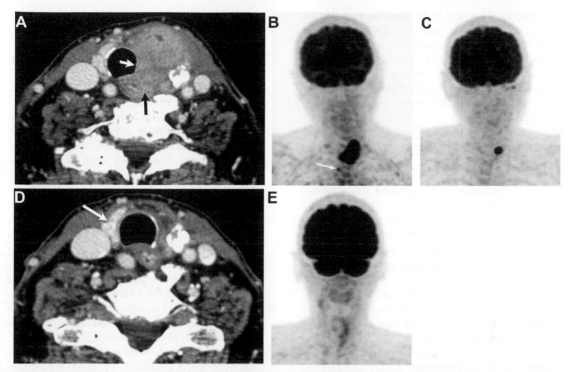

Fig. 2. A 79 year-old woman with left thyroid mass biopsy showing ATC. (*A*) Axial CECT shows locally invasive left thyroid tumor directly invading the trachea (*white arrow*) and esophagus (*black arrow*). Tumor infiltrates the tracheoesophageal groove and the midline structures are displaced toward the right. (*B*) Concurrent pretreatment F[18]-fluorodeoxyglucose (FDG) PET shows intense radiotracer uptake within the left thyroid tumor with central compartment nodal metastasis (*white arrow*). No lateral compartment lymphadenopathy. (*C*) Patient was initiated on dabrafenib and trametinib, and 3-month follow-up FDG-PET shows significant improvement in the left thyroid tumor. (*D*)Three-month follow-up CECT shows near resolution of the heterogeneously enhancing left thyroid tumor. Right thyroid lobe has a normal appearance (*white arrow*). (*E*) Patient was treated with left thyroid lobectomy and central neck dissection. FDG-PET obtained 2 months after resection and 5 months following initial diagnosis shows no residual metabolically active tumor in the neck.

SUMMARY

The understanding of the molecular drivers of thyroid cancer and the advances made in targeted therapies and immunotherapy have revolutionized the management of advanced thyroid cancer. Research has likely only scratched the surface when it comes to personalized therapies in this disease, targeting drivers such as *BRAF* mutations, and *RET* and *NTRK* fusions, as well as redifferentiation therapy. Future avenues of research could include antibody-drug conjugates, targeting other aspects of the immune microenvironment, and other pathway inhibitors.

CLINICS CARE POINTS

- Most patients with locally recurrent or metastatic DTC may be observed for a period of time as these patients often have indolent disease.

- All patients with ATC should be evaluated for BRAFV600E mutation with a rapid test, as upfront treatment with dabrafenib/trametinib should be initiated in stage IVC patients and unresectable stage IVB patients who may be candidates for neoadjuvant therapy followed by surgery.

DISCLOSURE

Dr M.E. Cabanillas has received grant funding from Eisai, Exelixis, Genentech, Merck and Kura. Advisory boards: exelixis, blueprint, Ignyta, Bayer and LOXO. The other authors have nothing to disclose.

REFERENCES

1. Cancer Genome Atlas Research Network. Integrated genomic characterization of papillary thyroid carcinoma. Cell 2014;159:676–90.

2. Pstrag N, Ziemnicka K, Bluyssen H, et al. Thyroid cancers of follicular origin in a genomic light: in-depth overview of common and unique molecular marker candidates. Mol Cancer 2018;17:116.

3. Landa I, Ibrahimpasic T, Boucai L, et al. Genomic and transcriptomic hallmarks of poorly differentiated and anaplastic thyroid cancers. J Clin Invest 2016; 126(3):1052–66.

4. Rao SN, Zafereo M, Dadu R, et al. Patterns of treatment failure in anaplastic thyroid carcinoma. Thyroid 2017;27:672–81.

5. Pozdeyev N, Gay LM, Sokol ES, et al. Genetic analysis of 779 advanced differentiated and anaplastic thyroid cancers. Clin Cancer Res 2018;24:3059–68.

6. Chen H, Luthra R, Routbort MJ, et al. Molecular profile of advanced thyroid carcinomas by next-generation sequencing: characterizing tumors beyond diagnosis for targeted therapy. Mol Cancer Ther 2018;17:1575–84.

7. Begum S, Rosenbaum E, Henrique R, et al. BRAF mutations in anaplastic thyroid carcinoma: implications for tumor origin, diagnosis and treatment. Mod Pathol 2004;17:1359–63.

8. Clayman GL, Agarwal G, Edeiken BS, et al. Long-term outcome of comprehensive central compartment dissection in patients with recurrent/persistent papillary thyroid carcinoma. Thyroid 2011;21:1309–16.

9. Chinn SB, Zafereo ME, Waguespack SG, et al. Long-Term Outcomes of Lateral Neck Dissection in Patients with Recurrent or Persistent Well-Differentiated Thyroid Cancer. Thyroid 2017;27:1291–9.

10. Brose MS, Nutting CM, Jarzab B, et al. Sorafenib in radioactive iodine-refractory, locally advanced or metastatic differentiated thyroid cancer: a randomised, double-blind, phase 3 trial. Lancet 2014; 384(9940):319–28.

11. Schlumberger M, Tahara M, Wirth LJ, et al. Lenvatinib versus placebo in radioiodine-refractory thyroid cancer. N Engl J Med 2015;372:621–30.

12. Cabanillas ME, Takahashi S. Managing the adverse events associated with lenvatinib therapy in radioiodine-refractory differentiated thyroid cancer. Semin Oncol 2019;46:57–64.

13. Blevins DP, Dadu R, Hu M, et al. Aerodigestive fistula formation as a rare side effect of antiangiogenic tyrosine kinase inhibitor therapy for thyroid cancer. Thyroid 2014;24:918–22.

14. Oishi K, Takabatake D, Shibuya Y. Efficacy of lenvatinib in a patient with anaplastic thyroid cancer. Endocrinol Diabetes Metab Case Rep 2017;2017. https://doi.org/10.1530/EDM-16-0136.

15. Iwasaki H, Yamazaki H, Takasaki H, et al. Lenvatinib as a novel treatment for anaplastic thyroid cancer: A retrospective study. Oncol Lett 2018;16:7271–7.

16. Brose MS, Cabanillas ME, Cohen EE, et al. Vemurafenib in patients with BRAF(V600E)-positive metastatic or unresectable papillary thyroid cancer refractory to radioactive iodine: a non-randomised, multicentre, open-label, phase 2 trial. Lancet Oncol 2016;17:1272–82.

17. Falchook GS, Millward M, Hong D, et al. BRAF Inhibitor Dabrafenib in Patients with Metastatic BRAF-mutant thyroid cancer. Thyroid 2014;25(1):71–7.

18. Shah MH, Wei L, Wirth LJ, et al. Results of randomized phase II trial of dabrafenib versus dabrafenib plus trametinib in BRAF-mutated papillary thyroid carcinoma. J Clin Oncol 2017;35.

19. Rothenberg SM, Daniels GH, Wirth LJ. Redifferentiation of Iodine-Refractory BRAF V600E-Mutant Metastatic Papillary Thyroid Cancer with Dabrafenib-Response. Clin Cancer Res 2015;21:5640–1.

20. Ho AL, Grewal RK, Leboeuf R, et al. Selumetinib-enhanced radioiodine uptake in advanced thyroid cancer. N Engl J Med 2013;368:623–32.

21. Groussin L, Clerc J, Huillard O. Larotrectinib-enhanced radioactive iodine uptake in advanced thyroid cancer. N Engl J Med 2020;383:1686–7.

22. Drilon A, Laetsch TW, Kummar S, et al. Efficacy of larotrectinib in TRK fusion-positive cancers in adults and children. N Engl J Med 2018;378:731–9.

23. Cabanillas ME, Drilon A, Farago AF, et al. Larotrectinib treatment of advanced TRK fusion thyroid cancer. Ann Oncol 2020;31(suppl_4) [abstract: 1916P].

24. Wirth LJ, Sherman E, Robinson B, et al. Efficacy of selpercatinib in RET-altered thyroid cancers. N Engl J Med 2020;383:825–35.

25. Subbiah V, Hu MI, Gainor J, et al. Clinical activity of the RET inhibitor pralsetinib (BLU-667) in patients with RET fusion+ solid tumors. J Clin Oncol 2020;38.

26. Subbiah V, Kreitman RJ, Wainberg ZA, et al. Dabrafenib and trametinib treatment in patients with locally advanced or metastatic BRAF V600-mutant anaplastic thyroid cancer. J Clin Oncol 2017;36(1):7–13.

27. Keam B, Kreitman RJ, Wainberg ZA, et al. Updated efficacy and safety data of dabrafenib (D) and trametinib (T) in patients (pts) with BRAF V600E-mutated anaplastic thyroid cancer (ATC). Ann Oncol 2018;29(suppl_8).

28. Wang JR, Zafereo ME, Dadu R, et al. Complete surgical resection following neoadjuvant dabrafenib plus trametinib in BRAF(V600E)-mutated anaplastic thyroid carcinoma. Thyroid 2019;29:1036–43.

29. Capdevila J, Wirth LJ, Ernst T, et al. PD-1 blockade in anaplastic thyroid carcinoma. J Clin Oncol 2020; 38:2620–7.

30. Lorch J, Barletta JA, Nehs M, et al. A phase II study of nivolumab (N) plus ipilimumab (I) in radioidine refractory differentiated thyroid cancer (RAIR DTC) with exploratory cohorts in anaplastic (ATC) and medullary thyroid cancer (MTC). J Clin Oncol 2020;38.

31. Cabanillas ME, Dadu R, Ferrarotto R, et al. Atezolizumab combinations with targeted therapy for anaplastic thyroid carcinoma (ATC). J Clin Oncol 2020;38(Suppl) [abstract: 6514].

Extrathyroidal Manifestations of Thyroid Disease: Graves Eye Disease

James Matthew Debnam, MD[a],*, Kirthi Koka, MS[b,c], Bita Esmaeli, MD[b]

KEYWORDS

- Graves disease • Graves eye disease (GED) • Extraocular muscles • Lacrimal gland

KEY POINTS

- Graves disease is an autoimmune disorder caused by antigens against the TSH receptor.
- Approximately 25% of patients with Graves disease develop Graves eye disease (GED).
- Signs of GED include extraocular muscle (EOM) enlargement, proptosis, and retro-orbital fat expansion.
- Compressive optic neuropathy (CON) develops from compression on the optic nerve by the EOMs and retro-orbital fat.
- Radiologic differential considerations include idiopathic orbital inflammation, immunoglobulin G4–related disease, lymphoma, metastasis, and infection.

INTRODUCTION

Under normal circumstances, the hypothalamic-pituitary axis regulates thyroid function. Low circulating levels of thyroid hormones, triiodothyronine (T3) and thyroxine (T4), cause the hypothalamus to release thyrotropin-releasing hormone (TRH). TRH stimulates thyrotrophs in the anterior pituitary gland to produce thyroid-stimulating hormone (TSH). TSH binds to a receptor in the thyroid gland that stimulates follicular cells to release T3 and T4 into the bloodstream.

Graves disease is an autoimmune disorder caused by the breakdown of immune tolerance to antigens against the TSH receptor. Circulating anti-TSH receptor (TSH-R) autoantibodies bind to the TSH receptor and stimulate the thyroid follicular cells to release T3 and T4. The increased T3 and T4 leads to thyrotoxicosis and autoreactive

lymphocyte deposition in the thyroid gland.[1] In addition, TSH-R, thyroglobulin (Tg), and thyroid peroxidase (TPO) have unusual properties that contribute to the breakdown of immune tolerance.[2]

Graves disease is more common in women, usually presenting between 30 and 60 years of age and has an annual incidence of 16 cases per 100,000 women and 3 cases per 100,000 men.[3] A genetic predisposition accounts for 79% of the risk for Graves disease and environmental factors account for approximately 21%.[4] Environmental risk factors include stress, smoking, radiation exposure, excessive iodine, vitamin D and selenium deficiency, and occupational exposure to Agent Orange. Epstein-Barr and Hepatitis C virus exposure also may play a role.[3]

Hyperthyroidism associated with Graves disease leads to symptoms such as fatigue,

No commercial or financial conflicts of interest and any funding sources for all authors.
a Department of Neuroradiology, The University of Texas MD Anderson Cancer Center, 1515 Holcombe Boulevard, Unit 1482, Houston, TX 77030-4009, USA; b Ophthalmic Plastic Surgery, The University of Texas MD Anderson Cancer Center, 1515 Holcombe Boulevard, Unit 1488, Houston, TX 77030-4009, USA; c Orbit, Oculoplasty, Reconstructive and Aesthetic Services, Sankara Nethralaya, No 18, College Road, Chennai 600006, India
* Corresponding author.
E-mail address: matthew.debnam@mdanderson.org

Neuroimag Clin N Am 31 (2021) 367–378
https://doi.org/10.1016/j.nic.2021.04.006
1052-5149/21/© 2021 Elsevier Inc. All rights reserved.

neuroimaging.theclinics.com

palpitations, anxiety, weight loss, sleep disturbance, heat intolerance, sweating, and polydipsia.[5,6] A nodular goiter may develop and cause dysphagia, a globus sensation, or orthopnea due to esophageal or tracheal compression. Thyroid dermopathy is a rare extrathyroidal manifestation of Graves with lesions that are characterized by thickened pigmented skin primarily involving the pretibial region.[7] Acropachy is another rare extrathyroidal manifestation of Graves disease that presents with clubbing of the fingers and toes.[8]

In approximately 25% of patients with Graves disease, an inflammatory condition affects the orbital soft tissues, named Graves eye disease (GED).[9,10] The exact mechanism of GED is unknown, however TSH-R antibodies appear to cross-react with antigens resulting in activation and infiltration by T lymphocytes with the release of inflammatory mediators.[11] The extraocular muscles (EOMs) are subsequently infiltrated with inflammatory cells such lymphocytes, eosinophils, macrophages, and plasma cells with an increased deposition of mucopolysaccharides. In chronic cases, fibrosis results from collagen deposition.[12]

GED is the most common disease of the orbits and affects all races. With an estimated prevalence between 0.5% and 2.0%, women are affected more often than men by a ratio of 4:1.[13] GED eye disease is sometimes the initial presentation, with Graves disease developing around the same time as GED. However, in patients with Graves disease, symptoms of GED usually manifest within 12 months of disease onset in approximately 70% of the patients.[14,15] Risk factors for the development of GED include a positive family history, stress, smoking, and uncontrolled hypothyroidism after radioactive iodine.[16]

Accurate and timely evaluation for the clinical features of GED is imperative in making an early diagnosis, identifying patients at high risk, and for medical and surgical treatment planning. Patients with GED present with a broad spectrum of clinical findings based on which orbital soft tissues are affected. Approximately 60% of patients develop mild symptoms, including fat expansion, inflammation of the levator muscle complex with resultant proptosis, eyelid retraction, and exposure of the globe.[17] Typically this pattern slowly evolves over months in the younger, predominantly female patients.[18] The remaining patients with GED experience enlargement of 1 or more the extraocular muscles leading to more significant symptoms. In these patients a biphasic disease course may occur with 6 to 18 months of a progressive phase followed by disease inactivity.

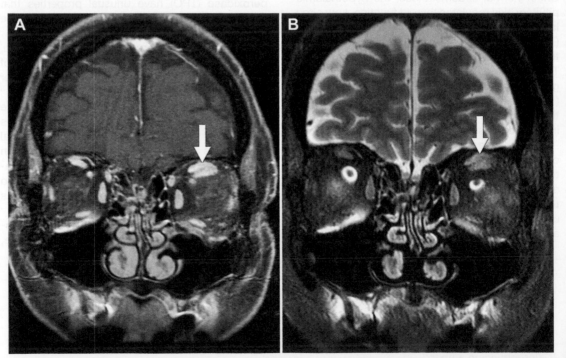

Fig. 1. MR imaging findings of thyroid eye disease. (A) Coronal T1 postcontrast sequence shows enlargement of the left levator complex with enhancement of the muscles (*arrow*). (B) Axial T2 sequence with T2 signal hyperintensity in the left levator complex (*arrow*).

Symptoms are more significant and include conjunctival and eyelid edema and congestion, restricted ocular movement with resultant diplopia, and optic nerve compression. These symptoms develop more rapidly, occur in an older population, and are often associated with a family history of GED and smoking.[18–20]

Retraction of the upper eyelid occurs in more than 80% of patients with GED and may be recognized by others.[21] A study by Davies and Dolman[22] found a correlation between upper eyelid retraction and an enlarged levator muscle complex, suggesting that antibodies most commonly affect this muscle. When present, retraction of the lower eyelid is associated with proptosis and inferior scleral show.

Proptosis occurs in GED from expansion of the retro-orbital fat and/or extraocular muscles. The combination of eyelid retraction and proptosis may lead to exposure of the cornea and GED symptoms, such as irritation of the corneal surface, excessive tearing, corneal ulceration, and even visual loss. Inflammation of the periorbital soft tissues may present with orbital discomfort at rest or with ocular movement, conjunctival injection and edema, and swollen red eyelids.

The commonly described order of frequency of EOM enlargement in patients with GED has been thought to be inferior rectus muscle as the most commonly affected EOM followed by the medial rectus, superior rectus, and then the lateral rectus muscles.[23–25] However, Dolman[18] described that the levator muscle complex is commonly involved in patients with GED and that significant involvement of the other EOMs is present in only one-third of patients. In 30% of patients with GED the levator muscle complex has been noted to be enlarged in isolation (Fig. 1).[22,26]

Clinically, EOM involvement may be associated with pain on eye movement, conjunctival infection, and edema of the body of the involved muscles. Progressive intermittent restriction of ocular motility occurs during the initial active inflammatory phase. Later, secondary fibrosis may lead to restriction of motility with diplopia and strabismus.[18]

A serious but relatively infrequent complication of GED is compressive optic neuropathy (CON), which occurs in approximately 6% of patients.[27] CON in patients with GED is thought to arise from compression of the optic nerve at the orbital apex by hypertrophied EOMs. The diagnosis is made clinically by detecting findings such as a relative afferent pupillary defect, dyschromatopsia, decreased visual acuity and a visual field defect, and decreased visual-evoked potentials.[28,29]

GRAVES EYE DISEASE GRADING SYSTEMS

Several classification schemes have been created to grade the severity of GED.

The NO SPECS Classification system grades GED-related signs and symptoms by assigning a Global Severity Score (Table 1). This system highlights the features of GED in order of the frequency of clinical presentations but does not include clinical activity or provide management guidelines.[30]

The European Group on Graves Orbitopathy scale is based on 3 categories of disease severity.[31] "Mild disease" is noted in patients with limited muscle involvement, mild eyelid retraction, and proptosis. Treatment may be conservative. "Moderate to severe disease" is present in patients with a greater degree of inflammatory

Table 1
NO SPECS classification

Classification	Signs and Symptoms (Grade)
0	No physical examination signs, asymptomatic
I	Only physical examination signs; for example, eyelid retraction
II	Soft tissue involvement (0: absent; a: minimal; b: moderate; c: marked)
III	Proptosis (0: absent, a: minimal, b: moderate, c: marked)
IV	Extraocular muscle involvement 0: absent a: minimal (limitation of gaze at extremes) b: moderate (restriction of motion without fixation) c: marked (fixation of globe)
V	Corneal involvement 0: absent a: minimal (corneal stippling) b: moderate (ulceration) c: marked (clouding, necrosis, perforation)
VI	Vision loss (optic nerve compression) 0: absent a: minimal (disc pallor; vision 20/20–20/60) b: moderate (disc pallor; vision 20/70–20/200) c: marked (blindness; vision <20/200)

Adapted from Werner SC. Classification of the eye changes of Graves' disease. Am J Ophthalmol 1969;68:646–8.

> **Box 1**
> **Clinical activity score**
>
> - Painful sensation behind globe
> - Pain with attempted gaze
> - Redness of eyelids
> - Injected (redness) conjunctiva
> - Chemosis (swelling of conjunctiva)
> - Eyelid inflammatory swelling
> - Caruncle inflammation
>
> *Data from* Mourits MP, Prummel MF, Wiersinga WM, et al. Clinical activity score as a guide in the management of patients with Graves' ophthalmopathy. Clin Endocrinol (Oxf) 1997;47:9–14.

change, proptosis (>25 mm), or restriction of motility impairing daily function. The treatment is often medical. "Very serious disease" refers to threatening conditions including CON and corneal ulceration, and may require surgical management.

The Clinical Activity Score (CAS) identifies patients with active GED who may benefit from treatment with immunosuppressive therapy through use of a summed binary scale (**Box 1**). Points are given for 7 periorbital soft tissue inflammatory signs and symptoms. On follow-up evaluation, additional points are recorded for increasing proptosis (2 mm or more), decreasing ocular motility (8° or more), or decreasing visual acuity. The CAS has a high predictive value for the outcome of immunosuppressive treatment for GED.[32] A CAS score of 4 or greater has an 80% positive predictive value and a 64% negative predictive value in assessing response to treatment with corticosteroids.[32]

The VISA system to assess GED is based on physical examination findings and patient symptoms. The system assesses 4 independent parameters including vision (V), inflammation (I), strabismus (S), and appearance (A). Each feature is considered and graded independently (**Table 2**). Patients with a moderate index score (<4 of 10) can be treated conservatively, whereas patients with higher index scores (>5 of 10) or showing evidence of progressive inflammation can be offered a more aggressive treatment regimen.[16,33]

DIAGNOSIS (CLINICAL)

The diagnosis of GED is based on 3 features of the disease.[34] Clinical findings include eyelid retraction with proptosis and limited orbital motility especially when the findings are bilateral. Abnormal T4 and TSH levels or a history of thyroid dysfunction help to confirm the diagnosis, although 10% of patients with GED are euthyroid at the onset of disease. Detecting TSH receptor antibodies has a high sensitivity for the presence of active Graves disease. Radiological studies including ultrasound, computed tomography (CT), and MR imaging may aid in the diagnosis.[35,36]

Table 2
VISA (vision, inflammation, strabismus, and appearance)

• Caruncle inflammation	0: Absent	1: Present
• Injected (redness) conjunctiva	0: absent	1: present
• Redness of eyelids	0: absent	1: present
• Diurnal variation of symptoms	0: absent	1: present
• Chemosis (swelling of conjunctiva)	0: absent	
	1: conjunctiva behind lid	
	2: conjunctiva beyond lid	
• Painful sensation behind globe		
At rest	0: absent	1: present
With gaze	0: absent	1: present
• Eyelid edema	0: absent	
	1: present without festoons (bags under eyes)	
	2: present with festoons	

Data from Barrio-Barrio J, Sabater AL, Bonet-Farriol E, et al. Graves' Ophthalmopathy: VISA versus EUGOGO Classification, Assessment, and Management J Ophthalmol. 2015;249125.

DIAGNOSIS (RADIOLOGIC)

Imaging is obtained in patients with GED to confirm the clinical diagnosis and to assess treatment response or interval worsening of disease. Approximately 90% of patients with GED have bilateral involvement even if the clinical manifestations are unilateral or asymmetric in terms of severity.[37]

CT and MR imaging demonstrate orbital pathology with exquisite detail. CT is better suited for the evaluation of bony structures, whereas MR imaging is preferred for soft tissue structures due to higher spatial resolution and ability to visualize edema. Both CT and MR imaging demonstrate findings of GED including swollen retro-orbital contents. In the acute phase, there is enlargement of the belly of the EOM with sparing of the tendinous insertions (Fig. 2), although on occasion the tendinous portion may be thickened. Imaging in the coronal plane is valuable in demonstrating EOM enlargement and compression on the optic nerve at the orbital apex (see Fig. 2). Hypodense areas in the EOMs also may be present from lymphocyte accumulation and deposition of mucopolysaccharides.[37] Cohen and colleagues[38] studied the Hounsfield unit (HU) density of the extraocular muscles to characterize fatty infiltration in patients with GED. They found a significantly lower mean HU density in patients with GED (−40.4 HU) compared with controls (−34.8 HU) (P = .048).

An increase in EOM volume, crowding of the EOM at the orbital apex, or effacement of the fat plane around optic nerve by the enlarged EOM can be seen with patients with signs of CON.[29,39–43] An increase in EOM volume can also lead to an increased intraocular pressure, proptosis, venous congestion, and periorbital edema.[44–47] Starks and colleagues[26] correlated visual field worst mean deviation (MD) in patients with CON with muscle group enlargement on orbit CT scans. They found that both increasing total muscle area and the area of the levator muscle complex correlated with worsening MD. In multivariate linear regression, the increasing area of the levator muscle complex remained a significant predictor of MD over total muscle area (P = .01).

Other findings on CT imaging in patients with GED include an increase of the orbital fat that may lead to stretching of the optic nerve, prolapse of the lacrimal gland, eyelid edema, and remodeling of the bony orbit (Fig. 3).[48,49]

On MR, the EOMs may appear T1 hyperintense due to fatty infiltration and T2 hyperintense from edema. Enhancement of the EOMs and enlargement also may be present (see Figs. 1 and 2). Dilation of the superior ophthalmic vein also may be noted. Several studies have used MR imaging to correlate MR imaging findings with severity of disease. Kvetny and colleagues[50] found a significant relationship between EOM thickness on T1-weighted sequences to disease severity using CAS as well as to the duration of disease activity. Tortora and colleagues[51] found a direct relationship between MR imaging signal intensity on the short tau inversion recovery (STIR) and T1 post-contrast- sequences and CAS. Higashiyama and colleagues[52] found that the signal intensity ratio of orbital fat on STIR correlated with disease severity.

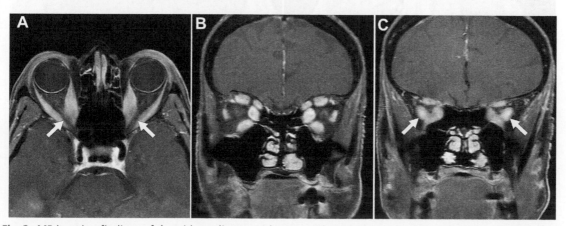

Fig. 2. MR imaging findings of thyroid eye disease with extraocular muscle involvement. (A) Axial T1 postcontrast sequence shows enlargement of medial and lateral rectus muscles with sparing of the tendinous insertions and associated mass effect on the optic nerves (arrows). (B) Coronal T1 postcontrast sequence through the mid orbit shows enlargement of the extraocular muscles. (C) Coronal T1 postcontrast sequence at the orbital apex shows muscle enlargement (arrows) with narrowing the space for the optic nerve to traverse.

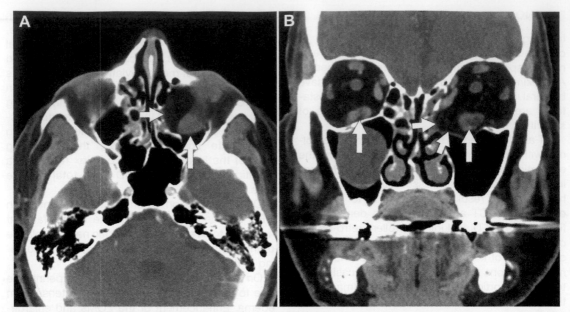

Fig. 3. CT findings of thyroid eye disease. (*A*) Axial postcontrast CT shows enlargement of the left inferior rectus muscle (*large arrow*) with excessive retro-orbital fat and postoperative changes from decompressive surgery (*small arrow*). (*B*) Axial postcontrast CT demonstrating enlargement of the left greater than right inferior rectus muscles (*large arrows*). Preponderance of retro-orbital fat is noted with postoperative change in the inferior medal orbital wall and the medial aspect of the orbital floor from decompressive surgery (*small arrows*).

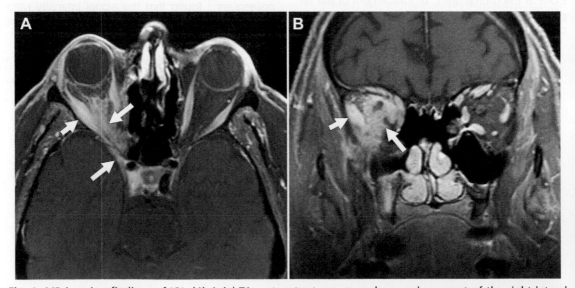

Fig. 4. MR imaging findings of IOI. (*A*) Axial T1 postcontrast sequence shows enlargement of the right lateral rectus muscle (*small arrow*) with disease involving the tendinous insertion and extending through the superior orbital fissure toward the cavernous sinus (*large arrow*). Additional disease is noted in the intraconal space (*large arrow*). (*B*) Coronal T1 postcontrast sequence demonstrates enlargement of the right lateral rectus muscle (*small arrow*) with disease in the intraconal space (*large arrow*).

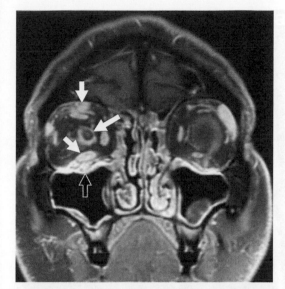

Fig. 5. MR imaging findings of IgG4-related disease. Coronal T1 postcontrast sequence with enlargement of the levator complex and inferior rectus muscles (*small arrows*). Enhancement is also present around the optic nerve (*large arrow*) and involving the infraorbital nerve (*black arrow*).

Radiologic signs of CON also can be evaluated on MR imaging. Dodds and colleagues[53] measured optic nerve diameter in patients with GED and CON, in patients with GED but without CON, and in control patients. They found that the narrowing of the optic nerve in patients with GED and CON was statistically significant when compared with those with GED but without CON. No significant difference was noted between patients with GED but without CON and control patients. The optic nerve narrowing most commonly affected the in the intraorbital apical and intracranial precanalicular segments. In addition, some of the patients with GED and CON showed optic nerve narrowing on MR imaging, whereas other patients in this group had proptosis with normal-appearing EOMs on MR imaging. This suggested to the investigators that compression on the optic nerve may also be related an increased volume of fat causing optic neuropathy.

RADIOLOGIC DIFFERENTIAL DIAGNOSIS

Several diseases affecting the EOMs are included in the radiologic differential diagnosis of GED.

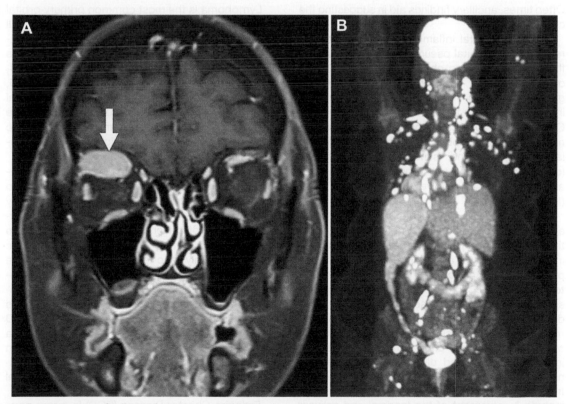

Fig. 6. MR imaging findings of lymphoma with orbital involvement. (*A*) Coronal T1 postcontrast sequence shows a well-circumscribed homogeneous enhancing mass in the superior orbit with involvement of the levator complex (*arrow*). (*B*) PET image demonstrates diffuse lymphadenopathy in the neck and throughout the body.

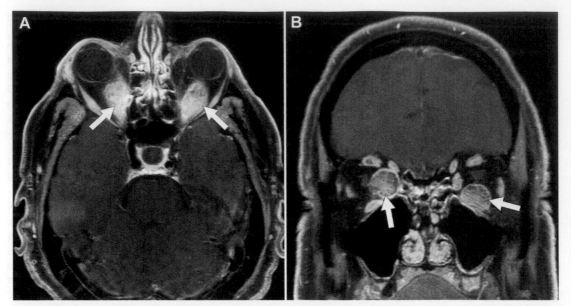

Fig. 7. MR imaging findings of gastrointestinal carcinoid tumor metastatic to the extraocular muscles. (*A*) Axial T1 postcontrast sequence and (*B*) coronal T1 postcontrast sequence showing heterogeneously enhancing lesions in the right medial and left inferior rectus muscles (*arrows*).

Often times, ancillary findings aid in suggesting the correct diagnosis.

Idiopathic orbital inflammation (IOI), previously referred to as orbital pseudotumor, is a painful inflammatory condition characterized by infiltration of polymorphous lymphocytes with varying degrees of fibrosis. Unlike GED, IOI can show involvement of the tendinous portion of the EOM. Other sites of IOI include the junction of the optic nerve and the globe (posterior scleritis), the lacrimal gland and surrounding soft tissues (dacryoadenitis), the optic nerve, retro-orbital fat, and extension to involve the cavernous sinus (Fig. 4).[54,55]

Immunoglobulin (Ig)G4-related disease is an autoimmune condition with diffuse or tumefactive lesions composed of lymphoplasmacytic infiltration with an abundance of IgG4-positive plasma cells with storiform fibrosis noted on histologic analysis.[56,57] Infiltration of the EOMs may spare the tendinous insertion and has been described to more commonly involve the lateral rectus muscle. Preseptal soft tissue swelling, orbital fat infiltration, and perineural involvement including the second division of the trigeminal nerve (V2) have also been described (Fig. 5).[58] In the head and neck, additional imaging findings include involvement of the lacrimal and salivary glands, pituitary glands, pachymeninges, and thyroid gland.[57]

Lymphoma is the most common primary orbital malignancy in adults and accounts for of 2% of all lymphomas and 8% to 15% extranodal non-Hodgkin's lymphomas.[59] The most common sites of involvement are the conjunctiva, eyelid, orbit, and lacrimal gland. When the EOMs are involved, the lesions are reported to usually be unilateral and painless with thickening of both the muscle and tendon. MR imaging features are nonspecific with T1 and T2 isointense signal and homogeneous enhancement (Fig. 6).[60]

Metastasis to the EOM is a common manifestation of orbital metastasis and in some series an enlarged EOM maybe seen in approximately 60% of cases of orbital metastases.[61] Approximately 58% of patients have been reported to have a known primary tumor at presentation. The most commonly reported primary tumors include breast cancer, cutaneous melanoma, and gastrointestinal tumors. Imaging findings of EOM metastasis include a nodular pattern of disease as opposed to the diffuse infiltration noted in GED (Fig. 7).[62,63] EOM metastases may occur at a delayed time from the primary disease and can involve single or multiple EOMs. Additional findings include lesions in the bony orbit or intracranial compartment.[63]

Erdheim-Chester Disease (ECD) is a rare non–Langerhein's-cell histiocytosis characterized by tissues infiltration with lipid-laden

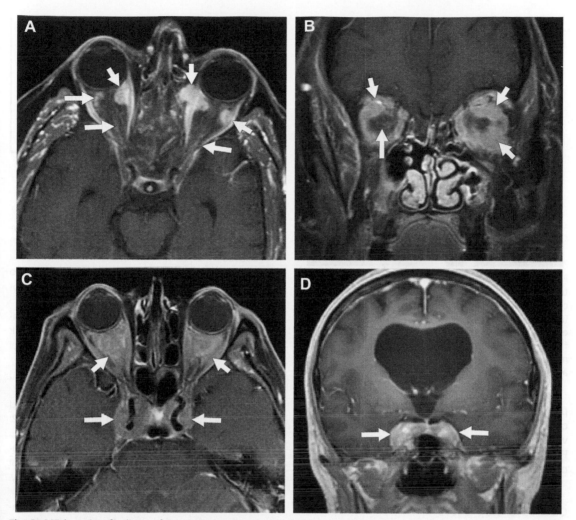

Fig. 8. MR imaging findings of ECD in 2 patients with orbital and intracranial involvement. (A) Axial T1 postcontrast sequence with multiple nodular enhancing foci involving the extraocular muscles (*small arrows*). Disease is also present in the retro-orbital space including around the optic nerves (*large arrows*). (B) Coronal T1 postcontrast sequence with enlargement of the left greater than right extraocular muscles (*small arrows*) and around the right optic nerve (*large arrow*). (C) Different patient. Axial T1 postcontrast sequence shows diffuse disease in the bilateral retro-orbital spaces (*small arrows*) and involving the cavernous sinuses (*large arrows*). (D) Coronal T1 postcontrast sequence demonstrates enlargement of the cavernous sinuses (*arrows*).

histiocytes.[64,65] Radiographically, ECD most commonly involves bone, where it presents as medullary sclerosis. In the head and neck ECD may involve the orbits (Fig. 8), hypothalamic-pituitary axis, brain parenchyma, and meninges, and the paranasal sinuses. Other sites of involvement elsewhere in the body include the mediastinum, pulmonary interstitium, retroperitoneum, and bony spinal column.[66–68]

Vascular etiologies of EOM enlargement include carotid-cavernous sinus fistula, arteriovenous malformations, venous angiomas, and dural-venous shunts. Vascular distention and increased venous pressure lead to EOM enlargement that may vary from a single unilateral EOM to uniform enlargement of the EOMs.[69]

Infection most commonly involves the medial recuts muscle via direct spread from the ethmoid sinus (Fig. 9).[70]

TREATMENT

In many cases, GED is self-limiting and improves spontaneously within 2 to 5 years.[11] In the early active phase, treatment including immunomodulators or radiotherapy may be required in an attempt to limit the destruction caused by the immune cascade.[71] Surgery may be indicated in the

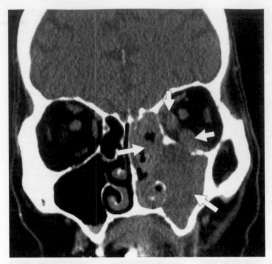

Fig. 9. CT findings of sinonasal infection causing extraocular muscle enlargement. Coronal CT without contrast demonstrating left sinonasal opacification (*large arrows*) consistent with infection. The infection extends through the laminal papyracea and orbital floor into the left orbit with enlargement of the medial and inferior rectus muscles (*small arrows*) and adjacent fat stranding.

postinflammatory phase for patient comfort, orbital cosmesis, and for preservation of function to halt vision loss from CON or corneal breakdown.[16] Recurrence of GED occurs in fewer than 10% of cases.[72]

CLINICS CARE POINTS

- Accurate and timely evaluation for the clinical features of Graves eye disease (GED) is imperative for early diagnosis, identifying patients at high risk, and for medical and surgical treatment planning.

- Classification schemes to grade the severity of GED include the NO SPECS Classification system, The European Group on Graves Orbitopathy scale, and the Clinical Activity Score (CAS).

- In the acute phase, there is enlargement of the belly of the extra-ocular muscle (EOM) with sparing of the tendinous insertions although occasionally the tendinous portion may be thickened. Imaging in the coronal plane is valuable in demonstrating EOM enlargement and compression on the optic nerve at the orbital apex.

- CT imaging findings in patients with GED include an increase of the orbital fat that

may lead to stretching of the optic nerve, prolapse of the lacrimal gland, eyelid edema, and remodeling of the bony orbit.

- On MR, the EOMs may appear T1 hyperintense due to fatty infiltration and T2 hyperintense from edema. Enhancement and enlargement of the extraocular muscles and dilation of the superior ophthalmic vein may also be present.

REFERENCES

1. Ferrari SM, Ruffilli I, Elia G, et al. Chemokines in hyperthyroidism. J Clin Transl Endocrinol 2019;17: 100196.
2. McLachlan SM, Rapoport B. Breaking tolerance to thyroid antigens: changing concepts in thyroid autoimmunity. Endocr Rev 2014;35:59–105.
3. Antonelli A, Ferrari SM, Ragusa F, et al. Graves' disease: Epidemiology, genetic and environmental risk factors and viruses. Best Pract Res Clin Endocrinol Metab 2020;34:101387.
4. Smith TJ, Hegedüs L. Graves' disease. N Engl J Med 2016;375:1552–65.
5. Devereaux D, Tewelde SZ. Hyperthyroidism and thyrotoxicosis. Emerg Med Clin North Am 2014;32: 277–92.
6. Boelaert K, Torlinska B, Holder RL, et al. Older subjects with hyperthyroidism present with a paucity of symptoms and signs: a large cross-sectional study. J Clin Endocrinol Metab 2010;95:2715–26.
7. Schwartz KM, Fatourechi V, Ahmed DD, et al. Dermopathy of Graves' disease (pretibial myxedema): long-term outcome. J Clin Endocrinol Metab 2002; 87:438–46.
8. Fatourechi V, Ahmed DD, Schwartz KM. Thyroid acropachy: report of 40 patients treated at a single institution in a 26-year period. J Clin Endocrinol Metab 2002;87:5435–41.
9. Lindgren AL, Sidhu S, Welsh KM. Periorbital myxedema treated with intralesional hyaluronidase. Am J Ophthalmol Case Rep 2020;19:100751.
10. Wei Y, Kang XL, Del Monte MA. Enlargement of the superior rectus and superior oblique muscles causes intorsion in Graves' eye disease. Br J Ophthalmol 2016;100:1280–4.
11. Cockerham KP, Kennerdell JS. Does radiotherapy have a role in the management of thyroid orbitopathy? View 1. Br J Ophthalmol 2002;86:102–4.
12. Glatt HJ. Optic nerve dysfunction in thyroid eye disease: a clinician's perspective. Radiology 1996;200:26–7.
13. Kendall-Taylor P, Perros P. Clinical presentation of thyroid associated orbitopathy. Thyroid 1998;8: 427–8.

14. Wiersinga WM, Smit T, van der Gaag R, et al. Temporal relationship between onset of Graves' ophthalmopathy and onset of thyroidal Graves' disease. J Endocrinol Invest 1988;11:615–9.

15. Noth D, Gebauer M, Müller B, et al. Graves' ophthalmopathy: natural history and treatment outcomes. Swiss Med Wkly 2001;131:603–9.

16. Dolman PJ. Grading severity and activity in thyroid eye disease. Ophthal Plast Reconstr Surg 2018;34:S34–40.

17. McKeag D, Lane C, Lazarus JH, et al. European Group on Graves' Orbitopathy (EUGOGO). Clinical features of dysthyroid optic neuropathy: a European Group on Graves' Orbitopathy (EUGOGO) survey. Br J Ophthalmol 2007;91:455–8.

18. Dolman PJ. Evaluating Graves' orbitopathy. Best Pract Res Clin Endocrinol Metabv 2012;26:229–48.

19. Kendler DL, Lippa J, Rootman J. The initial clinical characteristics of Graves' orbitopathy vary with age and sex. Arch Ophthalmol 1993;111:197–201.

20. Regensburg NI, Wiersinga WM, Berendschot TT, et al. Effect of smoking on orbital fat and muscle volume in Graves' orbitopathy. Thyroid 2011;21:177–81.

21. Frueh BR, Musch DC, Garber FW. Lid retraction and levator aponeurosis defects in Graves' eye disease. Ophthalmic Surg 1986;17:216–20.

22. Davies MJ, Dolman PJ. Levator muscle enlargement in thyroid eye disease-related upper eyelid retraction. Ophthal Plast Reconstr Surg 2017;33:35–9.

23. Feldon SE, Weiner JM. Clinical significance of extraocular muscle volumes in Graves' ophthalmopathy: a quantitative computed tomography study. Arch Ophthalmol 1982;100:1266–9.

24. Crisp M, Starkey KJ, Lane C. Adipogenesis in thyroid eye disease. Invest Ophthalmol Vis Sci 2000;41:3249–55.

25. Villadolid MC, Yokoyama N, Izumi M, et al. Untreated Graves' disease patients without clinical ophthalmopathy demonstrate a high frequency of extraocular muscle (EOM) enlargement by magnetic resonance. J Clin Endocrinol Metab 1995;80:2830–3.

26. Starks VS, Reinshagen KL, Lee NG, et al. Visual field and orbital computed tomography correlation in dysthyroid optic neuropathy due to thyroid eye disease. Orbit 2020;39:77–83.

27. Bartley GB. The epidemiologic characteristics and clinical course of ophthalmopathy associated with autoimmune thyroid disease in Olmsted County, Minnesota. Trans Am Ophthalmol Soc 1994;92:477–588.

28. Trobe JD, Glaser JS, Laflamme P. Dysthyroid optic neuropathy. Clinical profile and rationale for management. Arch Ophthalmol 1978;96:1199–209.

29. Neigel JM, Rootman J, Belkin RI, et al. Dysthyroid optic neuropathy. The crowded orbital apex syndrome. Ophthalmology 1988;95:1515–21.

30. Werner SC. Classification of the eye changes of Graves' disease. Am J Ophthalmol 1969;68:646–8.

31. Boboridis K, Perros P. General management plan. In: Wiersinga WM, Kahaly G, editors. Graves' orbitopathy: a multidisciplinary approach. Basel (Switzerland): Karger; 2007. p. 88–95.

32. Mourits MP, Prummel MF, Wiersinga WM, et al. Clinical activity score as a guide in the management of patients with Graves' ophthalmopathy. Clin Endocrinol (Oxf) 1997;47:9–14.

33. Barrio-Barrio J, Sabater AL, Bonet-Farriol E, et al. Graves' ophthalmopathy: VISA versus EUGOGO classification. Assessment, Management J Ophthalmol 2015;2015:249125.

34. Bahn RS, Kazim M. Thyroid eye disease. In: Fay A, Dolman PJ, editors. Diseases and disorders of the orbit and ocular adnexa. London: Elsevier; 2017. p. 219–34.

35. Polito E, Leccisotti A. MRI in Graves orbitopathy: recognition of enlarged muscles and prediction of steroid response. Ophthalmologica 1995;209:182–6.

36. Regensburg NI, Wiersinga WM, Berendschot TT, et al. Densities of orbital fat and extraocular muscles in graves orbitopathy patients and controls. Ophthal Plast Reconstr Surg 2011;27:236–40.

37. Rootman J. Diseases of the orbit: a multidisciplinary approach. Philadelphia: Lippincott; 1988. p. 143–240.

38. Cohen LM, Liou VD, Cunnane ME, et al. Radiographic analysis of fatty infiltration of the extraocular muscles in thyroid eye disease. Orbit 2020;2:1–6.

39. Feldon SE, Lee CP, Muramatsu SK, et al. Quantitative computed tomography of Graves' ophthalmopathy. Extraocular muscle and orbital fat in development of optic neuropathy. Arch Ophthalmol 1985;103:213–5.

40. Barrett L, Glatt HJ, Burde RM, et al. Optic nerve dysfunction in thyroid eye disease: CT. Radiology 1988;167:503–7.

41. Nugent RA, Belkin RI, Neigel JM, et al. Graves orbitopathy: correlation of CT and clinical findings. Radiology 1990;177:675–82.

42. Birchall D, Goodall KL, Noble JL, et al. Graves ophthalmopathy: intracranial fat prolapse on CT images as an indicator of optic nerve compression. Radiology 1996;200:123–7.

43. Goncalves AC, Silva LN, Gebrim EM, et al. Quantification of orbital apex crowding for screening of dysthyroid optic neuropathy using multidetector CT. AJNR Am J Neuroradiol 2012;33:1602–7.

44. Feldon SE, Muramatsu S, Weiner JM. Clinical classification of Graves' ophthalmopathy. Identification of risk factors for optic neuropathy. Arch Ophthalmol 1984;102:1469–72.

45. Peyster RG, Ginsberg F, Silber JH, et al. Exoph-thalmos caused by excessive fat: CT volumetric analysis and differential diagnosis. AJR Am J Roent-genol 1986;146:459–64.

46. Ohtsuka K. Intraocular pressure and proptosis in 95 patients with Graves ophthalmopathy. Am J Oph-thalmol 1997;124:570–2.

47. Gorman CA. The measurement of change in Graves' ophthalmopathy. Thyroid 1998;8:539–43.

48. Mafee MF, Miller MT. Computed tomography scan-ning in the evaluation of ocular motility disorders. In: Gonzalez CF, Becker MH, Flanagan JC, editors. Diagnostic imaging in ophthalmology. New York: Springer; 1988. p. 39–54.

49. Tan NYQ, Leong YY, Lang SS, et al. Radiologic pa-rameters of orbital bone remodeling in thyroid eye disease. Invest Ophthalmol Vis Sci 2017;58: 2527–33.

50. Kvetny J, Puhakka KB, Røhl L. Magnetic resonance imaging determination of extraocular eye muscle volume in patients with thyroid-associated oph-thalmopathy and proptosis. Acta Ophthalmol Scand 2006;84:419–23.

51. Tortora F, Cirillo M, Ferrara M, et al. Disease activity in Graves' ophthalmopathy: Diagnosis with orbital MR imaging and correlation with clinical score. Neu-roradiol J 2013;26:555–64.

52. Higashiyama T, Iwasa M, Ohji M. Quantitative anal-ysis of inflammation in orbital fat of thyroid-associated ophthalmopathy using MRI signal inten-sity. Sci Rep 2017;7:6–11.

53. Dodds NI, Atcha AW, Birchall D, et al. Use of high-resolution MRI of the optic nerve in Graves' oph-thalmopathy. Br J Radiol 2009;82:541–4.

54. Rothfus WE, Curtin HD. Extraocular muscle enlarge-ment: a CT review. Radiology 1984;151:677–81.

55. Yuen SJ, Rubin PA. Idiopathic orbital inflammation: distribution, clinical features, and treatment outcome. Arch Ophthalmol 2003;121:491–9.

56. Stone JH, Zen Y, Deshpande V. IgG4-related dis-ease. N Engl J Med 2012;366:539–51.

57. Cheuk W, Chan JK. IgG4-related sclerosing dis-ease: a critical appraisal of an evolving clinicopath-ologic entity. Adv Anat Pathol 2010;17:303–32.

58. Tiegs-Heiden CA, Eckel LJ, Hunt CH, et al. Immuno-globulin G4-related disease of the orbit: imaging features in 27 patients. AJNR Am J Neuroradiol 2014;35:1393–7.

59. Coha B, Vucinic I, Mahovne I, et al. Extranodal lym-phomas of head and neck with emphasis on NK/T-cell lymphoma, nasal type. J Craniomaxillofac Surg 2014;42:149–52.

60. Surov A, Behrmann C, Holzhausen HJ, et al. Lym-phomas and metastases of the extra-ocular muscu-lature. Neuroradiology 2011;53:909–16.

61. El-Hadad C, Koka K, Dong W, et al. Multidisciplinary management of orbital metastasis and survival out-comes. Ophthal Plast Reconstr Surg 2021. https://doi.org/10.1097/IOP.0000000000001939.

62. Lacey B, Chang W, Rootman J. Nonthyroid causes of extraocular muscle disease. Surv Ophthalmol 1999;44:187–213.

63. Alsuhaibani AH, Carter KD, Nerad JA, et al. Prostate carcinoma metastasis to extraocular muscles. Oph-thal Plast Reconstr Surg 2008;24:233–5.

64. Veyssier-Belot C, Cacoub P, Caparros-Lefebvre D, et al. Erdheim-Chester disease: clinical and radio-logic characteristics of 59 cases. Medicine 1996; 75:157–69.

65. Martinez R. Erdheim-Chester disease: MR of intraax-ial and extraaxial brain stem lesions. AJNR Am J Neuroradiol 1995;16:1787–90.

66. Drier A, Haroche J, Savatovsky J, et al. Cerebral, facial, and orbital involvement in Erdheim-Chester disease: CT and MR imaging findings. Radiology 2010;255:586–94.

67. Allmendinger AM, Krauthamer AV, Spektor V, et al. Atypical spine involvement of Erdhei77m-Chester disease in an elderly male. J Neurosurg Spine 2010;12:257–60.

68. Albayram S, Kizilkilic O, Zulfikar Z, et al. Spinal dural involvement in Erdheim-Chester disease: MRI find-ings. Neuroradiology 2002;44:1004–7.

69. Shafi F, Mathewson P, Mehta P, et al. The enlarged extraocular muscle: to relax, reflect or refer? Eye (Lond) 2017;31:537–44.

70. Towbin R, Han BK, Kaufman RA, et al. Postseptal cellulitis: CT in diagnosis and management. Radi-ology 1986;158:735–7.

71. Dolman PJ, Rath S. Orbital radiotherapy for thyroid eye disease. Curr Opin Ophthalmol 2012;23: 427–32.

72. Selva D, Chen C, King G. Late reactivation of thyroid orbitopathy. Clin Exp Ophthalmol 2004;32:46–50.

Parathyroid Imaging
Four-dimensional Computed Tomography, Sestamibi, and Ultrasonography

Sara B. Strauss, MD, Michelle Roytman, MD, C. Douglas Phillips, MD*

KEYWORDS

- Parathyroid adenoma • 4D-CT • Parathyroid scintigraphy • Dynamic contrast-enhanced 4D-MR

KEY POINTS

- Patients are referred for parathyroid imaging after the diagnosis of primary hyperparathyroidism has already been established, and therefore the radiologist's task is not to determine the diagnosis but to identify all operative candidate lesions.
- Knowledge of normal and variant parathyroid anatomy, including expected locations of ectopic superior and inferior glands, can aid in candidate lesion detection.
- Several imaging modalities are available for identification of parathyroid adenoma, including ultrasonography, scintigraphy, four-dimensional computed tomography (4D-CT), and magnetic resonance imaging, with various advantages and disadvantages to each.
- 4D-CT is particularly useful in the setting of multiglandular disease, ectopic parathyroid tissue, and in the setting of surgically refractory disease, and has supplanted other modalities such as ultrasonography and sestamibi as first-line imaging modality at many institutions.

INTRODUCTION

Primary hyperparathyroidism (PHPT) has an estimated prevalence of 1 to 7 cases per 1000 adults[1] and is more common in women than in men (female/male, 2–4:1) and white people in the fifth to seventh decade of life.[2] PHPT is most commonly a sporadic disease, but can be seen in the setting of multiple endocrine neoplasia type 1 or type 2a, familial hyperparathyroidism, and in patients with history of prior radiation to the neck. PHPT is associated with increased risk of pathologic fracture, nephrolithiasis, pancreatitis, peptic ulcer disease, cardiovascular disease, and neurocognitive disability. Diagnosis is rendered based on clinical and biochemical criteria, including increase of serum calcium and intact parathyroid hormone (PTH) levels in patients with normal renal function.[3] Hyperparathyroidism results most commonly from a parathyroid adenoma, a benign parathyroid tumor that causes high levels of PTH production.[4]

Surgical management remains the definitive cure for PHPT caused by parathyroid adenoma/hyperplasia and in the setting of tertiary hyperparathyroidism with autonomously functioning parathyroid tissue refractive to medical therapy. Surgical management is recommended even in asymptomatic patients who are low-risk surgical candidates.[3] Previously, wide-exposure, bilateral neck 4-gland exploration was the traditional approach to surgical management of PHPT, with a reported associated success rate of 95%.[5] In the setting of multiglandular disease, total parathyroidectomy with forearm or neck reimplantation or subtotal gland resection might be pursued. However, 4-gland exploration carries risks, including injury to the bilateral recurrent laryngeal nerves. Over the past 2 decades, more focused minimally

Department of Radiology, Weill Cornell Medical College, NewYork-Presbyterian Hospital, 525 E 68th Street, New York, NY 10065, USA
* Corresponding author.
E-mail address: Cdp2001@med.cornell.edu

Neuroimag Clin N Am 31 (2021) 379–395
https://doi.org/10.1016/j.nic.2021.04.007
1052-5149/21/© 2021 Elsevier Inc. All rights reserved.

invasive surgical strategies, including video-assisted parathyroidectomy, videoscopic parathyroidectomy, or unilateral open parathyroidectomy, have been increasingly used, and preoperative identification of a surgical target has become increasingly important.[6] Targeted surgery can be expanded to 4-gland exploration if intraoperative PTH assay does not show adequate decrease in PTH levels[7] (see Aditya S. Shirali's article, "Parathyroid Surgery: What the Radiologist Needs to Know," in this issue).

Several imaging modalities are available for identification of parathyroid adenoma. Historically, ultrasonography and technetium 99m-sestamibi single-photon emission computed tomography (SPECT)/computed tomography (CT) were the first-line modalities for preoperative evaluation for parathyroid adenoma. Although sensitivity and specificity of parathyroid scintigraphy and sonography are similar, combining their use has consistently been shown to more accurately predict the presence and location of solitary adenomas than either technique alone, up to 95% in some series.[8] Parathyroid scintigraphy is more advantageous than sonography in its ability to detect ectopic functional tissue, particularly when located within the mediastinum. However, both scintigraphy and sonography remain insensitive for the detection of multiglandular and/or ectopic disease or multiple parathyroid adenomas. Combined modalities have been shown to be only 60% sensitive in some case series of double parathyroid adenomas[9] and as low as 30% in multiglandular disease.[10]

Four-dimensional (4D) CT was introduced in the surgical literature in 2006 and, although parathyroid scintigraphy and sonography remain the most commonly used modalities, use of 4D-CT as a first-line study is increasing across institutions internationally.[11] A recent meta-analysis performed from 43 studies showed a pooled sensitivity and positive predictive value of 76.1% (95% confidence interval, 70.4%–81.4%) and 93.2% (90.7%–95.3%) for ultrasonography, 78.9% (64%–90.6%) and 90.7% (83.5%–96.0%) for sestamibi, and 89.4% and 93.5% for 4D-CT.[12] In terms of cost-effectiveness, ultrasonography followed by 4D-CT in patients with indeterminate initial examinations has been shown to be the least expensive model, followed by ultrasonography alone and 4D-CT alone.[13] Early application of magnetic resonance (MR) imaging to parathyroid detection was limited by poor spatial resolution, motion artifact, and incomplete fat saturation. However, MR imaging has been gaining traction because of increased use of higher field strength magnets, improved fat-saturation using chemical shift, parallel-imaging, and improved time-resolved techniques. Given concerns regarding radiation dose in scintigraphy and 4D-CT, this emerging option will likely continue to gain popularity.

This article describes strategies for imaging-based evaluation in the setting of PHPT, with a focus on identification of the single parathyroid adenoma and multiglandular disease.

EMBRYOLOGY/ANATOMY

The parathyroid glands play an important role in calcium homeostasis. Parathyroid tissue expresses calcium-sensing receptors, which detect calcium levels within the serum; when low levels of calcium are detected, parathyroid hormone is secreted, resulting in calcium release from bone, as well as increased calcium absorption and decreased phosphate absorption at the level of the kidney.[4] A normal parathyroid gland is not well seen on conventional imaging, measuring $5 \times 3 \times 2$ mm, and weighing between 40 and 50 mg.[14,15] PHPT results from a single adenoma in 75% to 85% of cases, 4-gland hyperplasia in 6% of cases, double adenoma in 4%, and rarely parathyroid carcinoma (1%).[2]

The paired superior glands and the thyroid both derive from the fourth pharyngeal pouch with a short migration distance, whereas the inferior glands and the thymus arise from the third pharyngeal pouch with a longer migration path.[5] Aberrant migration can result in ectopic parathyroid gland in adults, with a prevalence of 16% in patients with PHPT; this occurs more frequently with inferior compared with superior glands because of the longer migration path. Greater than 90% of superior glands are located deep to the superior thyroid between the cricoid and thyroid cartilages, but can be seen deep to the midthyroid (4%), above the thyroid (3%), retropharyngeal (1%), retroesophageal (1%), or even within the thyroid parenchyma (0.2%). The inferior glands are typically located adjacent to the lower pole of the thyroid (95%) but may be found more inferiorly in the neck or upper mediastinum within the thyrothymic ligament, carotid sheath, mediastinum, or within the thyroid parenchyma (28%). Rarely, the inferior glands fail to descend, and may be found above the level of the superior glands as high as the angle of the mandible.[15] The most common location for ectopic inferior parathyroid is the anterior mediastinum (Fig. 1), and most common ectopic location for superior parathyroid includes the tracheoesophageal groove and retroesophageal region[15] (Fig. 2). In the setting of ectopic parathyroid tissue, the most reproducible anatomic boundary

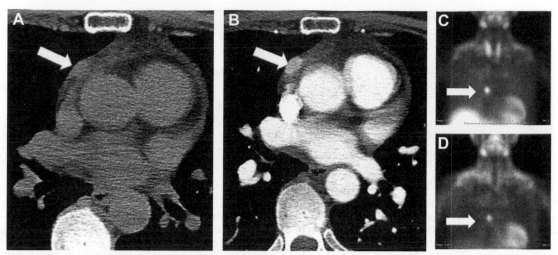

Fig. 1. Ectopic superior gland parathyroid adenoma in a 52-year-old woman with increased calcium and PTH levels. No lesion was visualized on ultrasonography. Axial noncontrast (*A*) and postcontrast (*B*) CT shows enhancing soft tissue in the anterior mediastinum (*white arrows*). Anterior [99mTc]-MIBI planar images at 10 minutes (*C*) and 2 hours (*D*) show activity in the anterior mediastinum (*white arrows*).

between superior and inferior parathyroid tissue is the plane of the recurrent laryngeal nerve within the tracheoesophageal groove, with the superior located posteriorly and inferior located anteriorly.[16] From 2.5% to 13% of individuals have supernumerary glands and 3% have fewer than 4 glands.[15] An understanding of normal and variant parathyroid anatomy helps to direct the search for abnormally functioning tissue in patients with PHPT (**Fig. 3**).

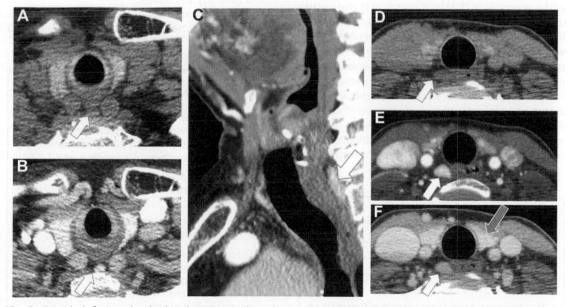

Fig. 2. Ectopic inferior glands. (*A–C*) Retroesophageal parathyroid adenoma: (*A*) axial noncontrast CT and (*B*) postcontrast CT shows retroesophageal soft tissue that is hypodense relative to thyroid on noncontrast images (*A, white arrow*) and hypoenhancing relative to thyroid on venous phase images (*B, white arrow*). (*C*) Sagittal postcontrast shows ovoid morphology (*white arrow*). (*D–F*) Tracheoesophageal groove parathyroid adenoma in a different patient: (*D*) axial noncontrast CT shows hypoenhancing soft tissue within the right tracheoesophageal groove (*white arrow*), with hyperenhancement on arterial phase imaging (*white arrow in E*) and washout on venous phase imaging (*white arrow in F*) relative to thyroid tissue (*gray arrow in F*).

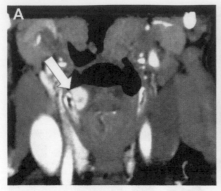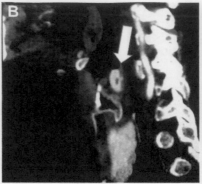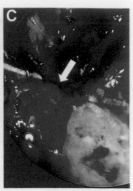

Fig. 3. Ectopic parathyroid adenoma within the right piriform sinus. Ovoid enhancing lesion is seen within the right piriform sinus on postcontrast coronal (*A*) and sagittal (*B*) reformatted images (*white arrows*). (*C*) The presence of ectopic parathyroid tissue was confirmed intraoperatively at the time of CO_2 laser-assisted excision (*white arrow*). Both the third and fourth pharyngeal pouches give rise to the pyriform fossa; early arrest of parathyroid descent with pharyngeal wall implantation is thought to underly this rare ectopy. (*Courtesy of* David Panush, MD, Hackensack University Medical Center and Bryan T. Ho, MD, Englewood Ear, Nose, & Throat, Englewood, NJ.)

IMAGING EVALUATION OF PRIMARY HYPERPARATHYROIDISM
Ultrasonography

Ultrasonography is the traditional first-line modality for evaluation of PHPT, and is highly accurate for identification of orthotopic parathyroid tissue, with improved spatial resolution compared with scintigraphy.[17] Ultrasonography is inexpensive, has no associated ionization radiation, and can be performed in conjunction with tissue sampling when appropriate (**Boxes 1** and **2**). It is particularly useful in chronic hypothyroidism, where a diffusely hypoattenuating thyroid gland makes comparison with parathyroid tissue challenging on CT. Classic parathyroid tissue shows homogeneous hypoechogenicity relative to thyroid on gray-scale imaging, with round, oval, or lobulated morphology with a craniocaudal long axis, and echogenic capsule (**Fig. 4**). More heterogeneous internal echoes may be present if there is fat, calcification, or hemorrhage. Internal cystic change might result in an anechoic lesion with increased through transmission. The presence of a fatty hilum and reniform morphology can help to differentiate between a lymph node and parathyroid adenoma in some instances. Color and power Doppler show a polar vessel with perilesional vascularity as the feeding vessel branches along the periphery of the gland[5,18] (see **Fig. 4**). Increased vascularity within an adenoma and a polar feeding vessel can serve as a useful tool in differentiating parathyroid adenoma from thyroid tissue.[19]

Several advanced sonographic techniques have been shown to help in diagnosis of parathyroid

---

Box 1
Ultrasonography: imaging protocols

- Patient is positioned supine, with hyperextended neck.

- Transducer: linear, high frequency, 12 to 15 MHz.

- B-mode scan area: from carotid bifurcation to thoracic inlet in longitudinal and from carotid to carotid in transverse. Full evaluation of thyroid is concurrently performed.

- Color or power Doppler (polar vessel identification).

Box 2
Ultrasonography: pearls and pitfalls

- Ultrasonography is particularly useful in setting of chronic hypothyroidism, when thyroid tissue is more likely to be isoattenuating relative to parathyroid adenoma on CT.

- Graded compression aids in differentiation between parathyroid gland from adjacent soft tissues.

- Asking patient to swallow helps to increase conspicuity of inferior glands.

- Three-dimensional ultrasonography enables multiplanar reformat views as well as volumetric reconstruction and has been shown to enhance sensitivity to detection of smaller parathyroid lesions.

- Fine-needle aspiration may be useful when location and morphology do not help to differentiate lymph node from parathyroid adenoma or for definitive diagnosis in the setting of possible intrathyroidal adenoma.

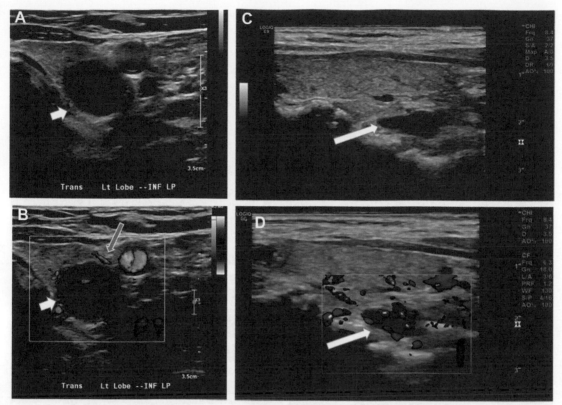

Fig. 4. Classic ultrasonography appearance of parathyroid adenoma. Transverse gray-scale images at the level of the left lower pole of the thyroid show a homogeneously hypoechoic lesion (*white arrow in A*). Peripheral vascularity (*white arrow*) and polar vessel (*gray arrow*) are shown on color Doppler (*B*). Right inferior parathyroid adenoma in a different patient shows a homogeneously hypoechoic lesion with lobulated contour and thin echogenic capsule (*white arrow in C*) with peripheral and intralesional vascularity on color Doppler imaging (*white arrow in D*).

adenoma. Sonoelastography is a new technique that evaluates the mechanical properties of tissue by analyzing response to acoustic energy, and can generate both qualitative as well as quantitative information regarding tissue stiffness and elasticity.[20] Several recent studies have shown that measures of lesion stiffness help to differentiate between parathyroid adenoma and benign and malignant thyroid lesions.[21] In addition, three-dimensional (3D) sonography has been shown to enhance sensitivity for parathyroid detection compared with two-dimensional ultrasonography, particularly in identification of smaller lesions (<500 mg).[22] Three-dimensional color Doppler can help to identify peripheral vascularity and polar vessel, allows accurate volume calculation, and enables tomographic viewing (**Fig. 5**).

Parathyroid Scintigraphy

Parathyroid scintigraphy is an important imaging modality for the identification and preoperative localization of hyperfunctioning parathyroid glands.[5,23–26] It is typically performed as a dual-phase, single-isotope (washout scintigraphic technique) examination using [99m]technetium-sestamibi (^{99m}Tc-MIBI), a radiopharmaceutical of choice because of its energy characteristics fit for imaging (140 keV photon energy; 6-hour physical half-life; low-energy parallel hole collimation) and avid localization in the mitochondria of parathyroid tissue[5,23–26] (**Boxes 3 and 4**). This examination relies on ^{99m}Tc-MIBI being taken up by both thyroid and parathyroid glands with a significant decrease of activity within normal thyroid tissue, typically within 30 minutes, and retention of radiotracer within pathologic parathyroid tissue (eg, parathyroid adenomas and parathyroid hyperplasia).[23] Normal physiologic ^{99m}Tc-MIBI uptake is identified within the salivary glands, thyroid gland, and myocardium[5,25] (**Fig. 6**). Asymmetric foci of increased radiotracer uptake may be seen on early images, representing abnormal parathyroid tissue superimposed on normal thyroid tissue.[23] Delayed images

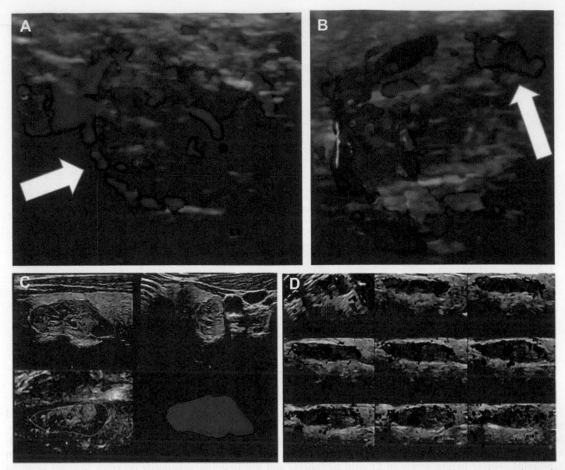

Fig. 5. Utility of 3D ultrasonography technique. Surface rendered view helps to show perilesional vascularity (*A, white arrow*) as well as feeding vessel (*B, white arrow*). Volume analysis can be performed in order to visualize surface geometry and calculate parathyroid volume (*C*). Tomographic ultrasonography imaging creates serial parallel slices of selected image thickness (*D*). (*Courtesy of* Susan Frank, MD, Montefiore Medical Center.)

are then acquired to identify foci of retained/hyper-concentrated radiotracer, characteristic of hyper-functioning parathyroid tissue. In addition to ^{99m}Tc-MIBI, ^{99m}Tc-tetrofosmin (^{99m}Tc-TETR) is an alternative radiotracer with parathyroid uptake and comparable imaging characteristics. Choice of imaging agent often depends on availability and experience of the interpreting physician.[23]

SPECT is often performed in conjunction with planar imaging.[5,23–27] SPECT generates 3D images using a 360° arc of image acquisition, analogous to CT images obtained from radiographs. A low-dose CT scan can be added to create a hybrid SPECT/CT scan, which further improves localization and sensitivity compared with planar imaging alone (**Fig. 7**). Three-dimensional imaging with SPECT/CT allows the differentiation of parathyroid activity from overlying thyroid tissue and may reveal small parathyroid adenomas not recognized

with planar imaging alone.[5,23–28] In 1 series, ^{99m}Tc-MIBI SPECT/CT was shown to precisely locate 90% of solitary adenomas, 73% of double adenomas, and 45% of hyperplastic glands.[28]

A single-phase dual-isotope (subtraction scintigraphic technique) examination can alternatively be performed using a radiotracer with parathyroid uptake, typically ^{99m}Tc-MIBI or ^{99m}Tc-TETR, in conjunction with a radiotracer without parathyroid uptake, typically ^{99m}Tc-pertechnetate or [123]I.[5,23–27] Using this technique, subtraction of the 2 acquisitions generates a parathyroid-only image (**Fig. 8**). Dual-isotope imaging may also be used in conjunction with single-isotope dual-phase imaging for problem-solving purposes.[23] Use of the subtraction scintigraphic technique may be particularly helpful in patients with history of thyroid disease (eg, goiter, thyroid adenomas, thyroid carcinomas) or thyroid surgery, in whom

---

Box 3
Parathyroid scintigraphy: imaging protocols

- The typical imaging protocol consists of intravenous administration of 20 mCi (740 MBq) ^{99m}Tc-MIBI.

- Initial acquisition of early anterior planar imaging at 5 to 30 minutes and delayed acquisition of anterior planar imaging at 1 to 3 hours (washout views).

- Routine large-field-of-view images, extending from the base of the jaw through the heart, should be performed because of the possibility of ectopic parathyroid adenomas.

- Sternal notch marker, as well as normal physiologic thyroid activity, can serve as anatomic landmarks for localization on planar images.

---

thyroid avidity may not decrease as rapidly as usual.

Positive parathyroid scintigraphy scans are associated with larger parathyroid glands (>500 mg in weight), whereas nonlocalizing or negative scans are often associated with low-weight parathyroid adenomas (<200 mg in weight) or multiglandular disease.[5,24,26] Size and cellularity of the glands, as well as level of parathyroid hormone, are known to affect sensitivity and specificity of parathyroid scintigraphy.[5,23,24,26] Potential sources of false-positive results in parathyroid scintigraphy include the presence of thyroid carcinomas or thyroid adenomas, which may

---

Box 4
Parathyroid scintigraphy: pearls and pitfalls

- Hyperfunctioning parathyroid tissue does not always persist on delayed ^{99m}Tc-MIBI imaging, so any avid foci seen on early images should be considered suspicious despite potential washout.

- Long-term use of some medications may result in nonvisualization of the thyroid with ^{99m}Tc-MIBI or ^{99m}Tc-tetrofosmin (^{99m}Tc-TETR) imaging; therefore, correlating scintigraphic patterns with clinical and surgical history is critical for the interpretation of parathyroid scintigraphy.

- If delayed ^{99m}Tc-MIBI or ^{99m}Tc-TETR images are inconclusive, patients can be reinjected with ^{99m}Tc-pertechnetate; if equivocal focus hyperconcentrates pertechnetate, it likely reflects a thyroid adenoma, whereas relative photopenia postpertechnetate indicates a parathyroid adenoma.

---

concentrate ^{99m}Tc-MIBI or ^{99m}Tc-TETR in a pattern typical of parathyroid adenomas.[5,23–26] Thyroid nodules have been reported to coexist with parathyroid adenomas in up to 30% of cases.[25] The presence of ectopic localization of radiotracer to the lateral aspect of the neck should raise the possibility of metastatic thyroid cancer. Other parathyroid mimics include physiologic asymmetric activity within the submandibular glands, as well as lymphadenopathy, sarcoidosis or Graves disease.[23,26] False-negative results occur when parathyroid adenomas show rapid washout similar to that of thyroid tissue; therefore, any avid foci seen on early images should be considered suspicious despite potential washout.[23] Other limitations of parathyroid scintigraphy include the potential for motion degradation caused by the length of time required for study acquisition, increased cost compared with sonography or 4D-CT, and increased radiation exposure, with a corresponding estimated increased lifetime attributable cancer risk of 0.19%.[26]

Although ^{99m}Tc-MIBI washout and/or subtraction scintigraphy with concurrent SPECT/CT are established techniques for parathyroid adenoma detection, there is emerging literature regarding use of PET for parathyroid adenoma detection. Several PET radiotracers have been described, including ^{18}F-fluorocholine, ^{18}F-fluorodeoxyglucose, ^{11}C-methionine, and ^{11}C-choline; however, no ideal PET tracer has emerged.[28,29] A case series using ^{11}C-choline PET/CT showed it to be a promising tool for localization of parathyroid adenomas, with advantages including a shorter acquisition time and clearer image interpretation compared with existing methods.[29] However, its short half-life (approximately 20 minutes) limits widespread use.[29] A case series using ^{18}F-fluorocholine PET/CT showed its ability to localize enlarged parathyroid tissue, with an optimal scan time of 1 hour after radiotracer administration.[30] ^{68}Ga-PSMA (prostate-specific membrane antigen) PET/CT has also been reported to incidentally detect a parathyroid adenoma in a case report.[31] Although PET/CT may serve as a problem-solving tool in the evaluation of false-negative or discordant results, further evaluation is required to identify the optimal radiotracers and protocols for its use.[26]

Four-Dimensional Computed Tomography

Four-dimensional CT was initially introduced in the surgical literature in 2006, and has subsequently been shown to have high diagnostic accuracy for both identification of parathyroid disease and lateralization of single-gland disease.[32,33] Four-dimensional CT has improved diagnostic accuracy

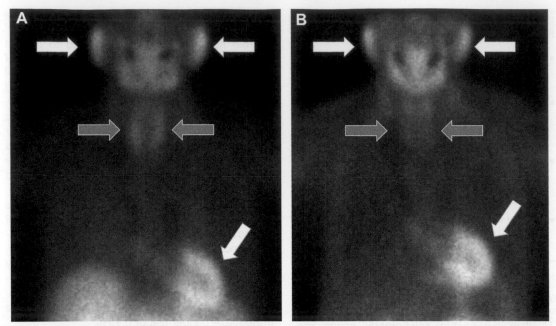

Fig. 6. Normal physiologic uptake. Early (*A*) and delayed (*B*) anterior ⁹⁹ᵐTc-MIBI planar images show normal physiologic uptake within the salivary glands and myocardium (*white arrows*). Thyroid gland shows interval decrease in activity on delayed scan (*gray arrows*).

compared with ultrasonography and scintigraphy[12,34–37] for both single-gland and multigland disease, without improvement in diagnostic performance when both modalities were combined.[38] Four-dimensional CT is particularly useful in the setting of multiglandular disease, previously operated necks, recurrent PTHP,[39,40] and in the absence of ultrasonography or sestamibi diagnosis, and is increasingly used as part of routine

preoperative evaluation at many institutions.[11,37,41,42]

Four-dimensional CT is a multiphase protocol that usually consists of limited noncontrast acquisition followed by arterial and venous phase postcontrast acquisitions, with multiplanar reconstruction and coverage extending from the maxilla to the carina (**Boxes 5** and **6**). The fourth dimension refers to changes in perfusion over time. There is discussion

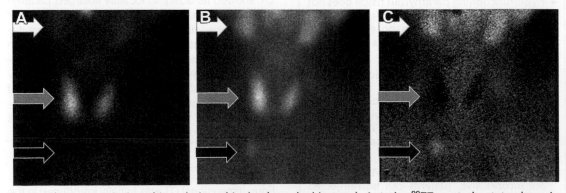

Fig. 7. Subtraction scintigraphic technique (single-phase dual isotope). Anterior ⁹⁹ᵐTc-pertechnetate planar image (*A*) shows homogeneous distribution of radiotracer throughout the normally positioned thyroid gland (*gray arrow*). Anterior ⁹⁹ᵐTc-MIBG planar image (*B*) shows homogeneous radiotracer uptake within the thyroid gland, with an additional discrete focus identified in the upper right chest (*black arrow*). Subtraction image (*C*) shows complete subtraction of the thyroid gland (*gray arrow*) with a persistent focus in the right upper chest, suggestive of ectopic parathyroid tissue. Normal physiologic uptake is seen in the salivary glands (*white arrows*).

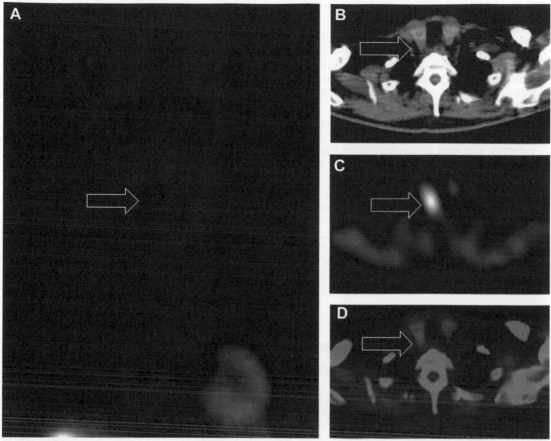

Fig. 8. SPECT/CT. Delayed anterior ^{99m}Tc-MIBI planar image (*A*) shows persistent activity overlying the superior right lobe of the thyroid (*black arrow*). CT (*B*), SPECT (*C*), and fused SPECT/CT (*D*) through the superior right lobe of the thyroid show a posterior 1.1-cm soft tissue nodule correlating to the region of ^{99m}Tc-MIBI activity, suspicious for a parathyroid adenoma.

in the literature regarding the ideal number of imaging acquisition time points, with various arguments made for anywhere from 2 up to 4 time points at 30 to 90 seconds after contrast injection.[33,39,42–45] Approximately half of institutions use a 3-phase protocol, with the remaining using 2 or 4 phases.[11] In addition, other mechanisms to further improve CT imaging can be performed, including placing a towel between the scapulae or use of footboard or shoulder strap to prevent beam-hardening artifact.

Candidate parathyroid lesions are evaluated relative to normal thyroid tissue with the goal being to differentiate a potential lesion from lymph nodes and thyroid tissue. Both orthotopic and known ectopic locations should be carefully interrogated. A classic parathyroid adenoma is hypoattenuating relative to the thyroid on noncontrast sequence, hyperattenuating relative to thyroid on arterial phase images, and hypoattenuating relative to the thyroid on venous phase images (**Fig. 9**). This

pattern mirrors parathyroid staining described in the angiographic literature.[46] In reality, the classic

---

Box 5

Four-dimensional computed tomography: imaging protocols

- Coverage: mandibular teeth to carina.

- Injection of 120 mL of 300 mg iodine/mL at 4 mL/s, followed by a 40-mL saline flush, arterial phase (25 seconds after injection), venous phase (30 delay from arterial phase).

- Thickness: 1.25 mm, at 1-mm intervals.

- Tube voltage 120 kVp; automatic modulation for tube current 150 to 300 mA.

- Pitch of 0.984:1.

- Display field of view of 18 cm for precontrast, 25 cm for postcontrast.

enhancement pattern is seen in only 20% of cases and may be related to lesion size; larger lesions (>1 cm^3) are more likely to show classic enhancement kinetics compared with smaller lesions (<1 cm^3).[47] Most parathyroid adenomas (57% of lesions) do not show arterial phase hyperenhancement relative to thyroid, but do show washout on venous phase, and 22% only show hypoattenuation relative to thyroid on noncontrast images, without hyperenhancement on arterial phase or washout on venous phase.[48] Nevertheless, a recent meta-analysis showed that the addition of a third phase resulted in a modest increase in performance sensitivity (80%) compared with 76% with 2 phases.[49] Dual energy CT may also be used to decrease dose by up to 50%.[50] Four-dimensional CT has been shown to be up to 93% accurate for lateralization of single-gland disease[33] and to have up to 70% sensitivity for quadrant identification.[34]

Consistent with previous descriptions of the appearance of parathyroid adenomas on catheter-directed angiography,[51] the presence of

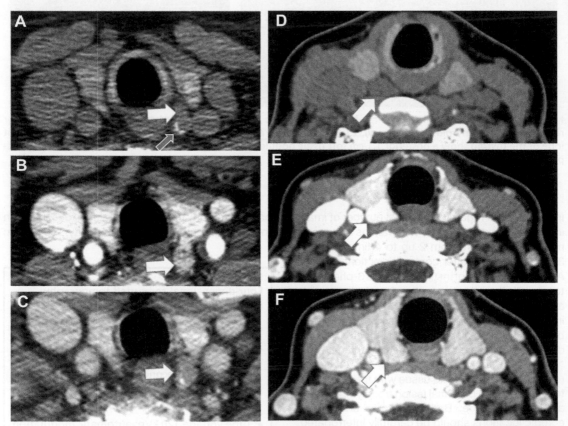

Fig. 9. Axial noncontrast (A), arterial phase (B), and venous phase (C) CT images at the level of the thyroid gland show robust arterial phase enhancement (*white arrow in B*) with washout on venous phase images (*white arrow in C*). Note calcification along posterior aspect of the lesion (*gray arrow in A*), which can contribute to heterogenous appearance on ultrasonography and MR. Classic (type A) parathyroid adenoma enhancement pattern in a different patient shows hypoattenuation relative to thyroid gland on noncontrast CT (*white arrow* in D), hyperenhancement on arterial phase (*white arrow* in E), and washout on venous phase (*white arrow* in F).

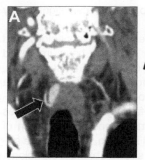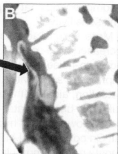

Fig. 10. Coronal (*A*) and oblique (*B*) reformatted images show a polar vessel (*black arrows*) in association with a right lower pole parathyroid adenoma.

a polar vessel, or prominent artery or draining vein, often in conjunction with a hypertrophied inferior thyroidal artery, might further point toward parathyroid adenoma and is seen in approximately two-third of cases, often with corresponding robust arterial phase enhancement[52] (Fig. 10). Adenomas tend to be ovoid or round, although may also be more oblong or pyramidal. Internal cystic change, calcification (as in Fig. 9), or fat may be variably present. The presence of a fat plane between a candidate lesion and the thyroid gland does not necessarily differentiate between thyroid nodule and parathyroid adenoma, because parathyroid tissue can be subcapsular (Fig. 11) and there can be extracapsular sequestration of thyroid tissue.[53]

Multiglandular disease is seen in 10% to 30% patients with PHPT[2] and is suspected on 4D-CT either when multiple candidate lesions are identified or,

importantly, when no lesions are identified. Likelihood of multiglandular disease can be predicted based on a composite multiglandular disease score developed by Sepahdari and colleagues,[54] which combines 4D-CT and clinical parameters and includes (1) lesion size, (2) total lesion number, and (3) Wisconsin Index (serum calcium in milligrams per deciliter) times parathyroid hormone levels (picograms per mL). In general, multiglandular disease lesions are smaller (mean size of 7.5 mm) than single-gland disease (mean size of 11.3 mm)[55] and should be considered in the setting of multiple small lesions (>7 mm), or when no candidate lesions are identified. Recently, Yeh and colleagues[56] found excellent reliability, moderate agreement, and positive correlation between estimated adenoma weight by multiplying the length, width, and height measurements (millimeters) by 0.63 mg/mm^3, and showed that estimated weight of greater than 50 mg distinguished parathyroid adenoma from normal glandular tissue.[56]

Although the effective dose for 4D-CT is greater than that of scintigraphy (28 mSv vs 12 mSv in study performed by Hoang and colleagues[11]), given that the typical patient with PHPT is a middle-aged woman, the lifetime attributable risk of cancer greater than baseline is only minimally increased (0.52% for 4D-CT compared with 0.19% for scintigraphy). Nevertheless, given the higher thyroid radiation dose compared with sestamibi with single-photon emission, use of this tool in patients of younger age might require consideration.[57] Because of the increased radiation dose, recent studies have suggested

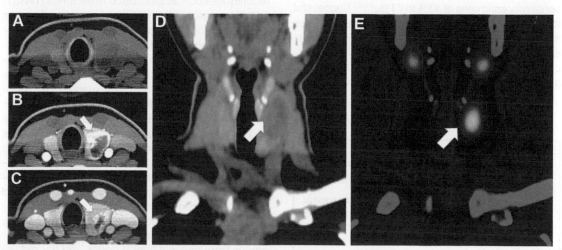

Fig. 11. Intracapsular parathyroid adenoma in a 55-year-old woman with PHPT. 4D-CT images (*A–C*) show a heterogeneous lesion within the left lobe of the thyroid; note arterial phase enhancement and washout in the peripheral, solid component of the lesion (*white arrows in B and C*). Low-dose CT (*D*) and fused SPECT-CT (*E*) show ^{99m}Tc-MIBI activity at the site of the lesion, which was confirmed to be intrathyroidal parathyroid adenoma at the time of hemithyroidectomy, with decrease in intraoperative PTH level from 273.4 to 30.3 pg/mL.

eliminating the noncontrast phase of the 4D-CT examination[48]; however, that subset of lesions do not show typical enhancement pattern on arterial and venous phases and are therefore only identified on the noncontrast portion of the examination.[48]

Magnetic Resonance Imaging and Dynamic Contrast-Enhanced Perfusion

Given the radiation exposure associated with 4D-CT and the associated increased lifetime attributable cancer risk in younger populations, MR imaging presents an appealing alternative (Boxes 7 and 8). Historically, MR imaging has been viewed as suboptimal for evaluation of parathyroid adenoma because of lower spatial resolution and potential for motion artifact related to swallowing,[58–60] with sensitivity estimates of 43% to 71%.[61,62] Successful identification of parathyroid adenoma requires robust fat-suppression techniques in order to differentiate lesion from adjacent soft tissues and to increase conspicuity given that parathyroid adenomas are typically lipid-poor lesions; as such,

inhomogeneous fat suppression can significantly limit sensitivity.[63]

More recent advances in MR technology and increased use of 3-T magnets have improved signal-to-noise and contrast-to-noise ratios, improving sensitivity for parathyroid adenoma detection, albeit with moderate success.[63] Chemical shift–based water-fat separation techniques have allowed more homogeneous suppression of fat. On conventional MR imaging, a parathyroid adenoma most commonly shows oblong morphology, hyperintensity on T2-weighted imaging, intermediate signal intensity on T1-weighted imaging, and avid enhancement on postcontrast sequences[64] (Fig. 12). India ink artifact on out-of-phase imaging can be leveraged to define a cleavage plane between parathyroid adenoma and adjacent tissues.[65] A subset of lesions may also show a marbled appearance on fat-suppressed T2- weighted sequences, which may reflect internal hemorrhage, cholesterol clefts, or fibrosis, and can help to differentiate adenoma from lymph node.[65] Robust T2 hyperintensity has been shown to be more reliable in identification of parathyroid adenoma than arterial phase enhancement, the latter of which has been described as only variably present on postcontrast MR imaging sequences.[65,66] As with 4D-CT, the presence of multiple candidate lesions suggests multiglandular disease (Fig. 13).

Dynamic 4D-MR imaging has been developed based on improvements in spatial and temporal resolution in application of time-resolved techniques and is an emerging technique in parathyroid adenoma imaging.[67–70] Time-resolved imaging techniques such as stochastic trajectories (TWIST) and time-resolved imaging of contrast kinetics (TRICKs) perform frequent sampling of the center of k-space, allowing high temporal and spatial resolution over the course of intravenous contrast material transit.[63] Parallel imaging techniques such as controlled aliasing in parallel imaging results in higher acceleration (CAIPIRINHA) have further opened avenues toward decreased imaging time and improved adenoma detection.[67,71,72] Nael and colleagues[71] performed a multiparametric quantitative analysis using dynamic contrast-enhanced (DCE) perfusion MR in parathyroid adenoma, and found that time to peak, wash-in, and washout differentiated between parathyroid adenoma, lymph node, and thyroid with high sensitivity and specificity for differentiating parathyroid adenomas from cervical lymph nodes and thyroid tissue.[71] Using this technique, the group showed a sensitivity of 100% for side and 92% for quadrant for single-gland disease, and 74% for the side and 77% for the quadrant for multiglandular

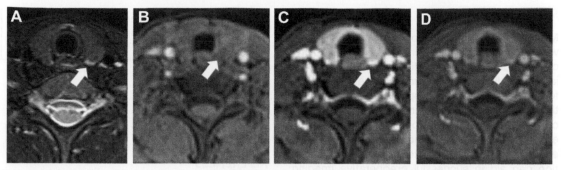

Fig. 12. MR imaging appearance of parathyroid adenoma. Axial fat-suppressed T2-weighted sequence shows a T2 hyperintense lesion posterior to the left lobe of the thyroid (*white arrow in A*). Fat-suppressed T1-weighted sequences without contrast (*B*), arterial phase (*C*), and venous phase (*D*) show intermediate signal intensity on T1-weighted sequence (*white arrow* in *B*) robust arterial phase enhancement (*white arrow in C*) with washout on delayed images (*white arrow in D*). (*Courtesy of* Kambiz Nael, MD, UCLA Medical Center.)

disease.[72] The investigators attribute their success to use of high-temporal-resolution DCE (6 seconds) and incorporation of Dixon technique for fat suppression. Although not yet widely used, dynamic 4D-MR imaging presents as an emerging approach for PHPT imaging.

Intraoperative Imaging

With the increasing use of small ultrasonography devices, often as a physical diagnosis tool and as a routine instrument in some clinical practices (as in active head and neck practices), more head and neck surgeons are facile with ultrasonography and have incorporated this as an adjunct operative tool. Using a small probe in a sterile cover, real-time sonography can be used to further refine the small incision used for minimally invasive parathyroid surgery. If surgeons are not confident in their own ultrasonography technique, a technologist or physician can attend the surgery to assist in the localization.[73] Parathyroid scintigraphy can also be used for intraoperative parathyroid localization, a technique termed radioguided parathyroidectomy.[26] In this method, ^{99m}Tc-MIBI is intravenously injected approximately 2 hours before surgery with intraoperative use of a small gamma probe to localize the parathyroid adenoma.[9] Small nuclear medicine detectors with sterile covers can accurately increase the success in accessing parathyroid adenomas that show significant uptake of the radionuclide. Intraoperative detection has been reported to be a safe and reliable adjunct to preoperative imaging localization and intraoperative monitoring.[26]

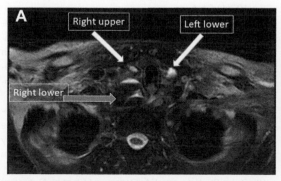
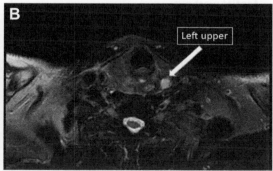

Fig. 13. Multiglandular hyperplasia with hemorrhage in a 71-year-old man. Axial fat-suppressed T2-weighted images show 4-gland enlargement (*A and B*). The right lower gland shows internal hematocrit levels, compatible with hemorrhage (*gray arrow in A*). (*Courtesy of* Deborah R. Shatzkes, MD, Hofstra Northwell School of Medicine, Lenox Hill Hospital.)

SUMMARY

Multiple modalities exist for evaluation of PHPT, with various advantages in terms of sensitivity, cost-effectiveness, and radiation exposure. Familiarity with limitations of each approach can help formulate a diagnostic approach, particularly in the setting of multiglandular disease, variant anatomy, and the previously operated neck. Knowledge of normal parathyroid anatomy as well as expected locations for ectopic parathyroid location can aid in successful preoperative imaging evaluation for parathyroid adenoma and parathyroid hyperplasia, regardless of technique. Successful preoperative localization of candidate parathyroid tissue supports minimally invasive techniques and avoids the potentially more morbid 4-gland exploration.

CLINICS CARE POINTS

- Patients are referred for parathyroid imaging after the diagnosis of PHPT has already been established, and therefore the radiologist's task is not to determine the diagnosis but to identify all operative candidates in order to potentially avoid 4-gland exploration.

- Evaluation of all possible sites for parathyroid tissue, including potentially ectopic superior and inferior glands, is critical to complete evaluation; the most common ectopic locations are the tracheoesophageal groove and retroesophageal region for superior parathyroid and anterior mediastinum for inferior parathyroid.

- Hyperfunctioning parathyroid tissue does not always persist on delayed 99mTc-MIBI imaging, so any avid foci seen on early images should be considered suspicious despite potential washout.

- Three-dimensional ultrasonography enables multiplanar reformat views as well as volumetric reconstruction and has been shown to enhance sensitivity to detection of smaller parathyroid lesions.

- Four-dimensional CT is an important tool in the setting of multiglandular disease, ectopic parathyroid tissue, and surgically refractory PHPT and has increasingly been incorporated as part of routine evaluation.

- Classic enhancement pattern on 4D-CT is seen in only 20% of cases, and careful evaluation of all candidates showing hypoattenuation relative to thyroid tissue on noncontrast phase images must be performed.

- DCE perfusion has been shown to help differentiate between lymph node and thyroid nodules on MR imaging.

DISCLOSURE

The authors have nothing to disclose.

REFERENCES

1. Yeh MW, Ituarte PH, Zhou HC, et al. Incidence and prevalence of primary hyperparathyroidism in a racially mixed population. J Clin Endocrinol Metab 2013;98(3):1122–9.

2. Ruda JM, Hollenbeak CS, Stack BC Jr. A systematic review of the diagnosis and treatment of primary hyperparathyroidism from 1995 to 2003. Otolaryngol Head Neck Surg 2005;132(3):359–72.

3. Bilezikian JP, Khan AA, Potts JT Jr, Hyperthyroidism TIWotMoAP. Guidelines for the management of asymptomatic primary hyperparathyroidism: summary statement from the third international workshop. J Clin Endocrinol Metab 2009;94(2):335–9.

4. Peissig K, Condie BG, Manley NR. Embryology of the parathyroid glands. Endocrinol Metab Clin North Am 2018;47(4):733.

5. Johnson NA, Tublin ME, Ogilvie JB. Parathyroid imaging: technique and role in the preoperative evaluation of primary hyperparathyroidism. Am J Roentgenol 2007;188(6):1706–15.

6. Sackett WR, Barraclough B, Reeve TS, et al. Worldwide trends in the surgical treatment of primary hyperparathyroidism in the era of minimally invasive parathyroidectomy. Arch Surg 2002; 137(9):1055–9.

7. Beland MD, Mayo-Smith WW, Grand DJ, et al. Dynamic MDCT for localization of occult parathyroid adenomas in 26 patients with primary hyperparathyroidism. Am J Roentgenology 2011; 196(1):61–5.

8. Lumachi F, Zucchetta P, Marzola M, et al. Advantages of combined technetium-99m-sestamibi scintigraphy and high-resolution ultrasonography in parathyroid localization: comparative study in 91 patients with primary hyperparathyroidism. Eur J Endocrinol 2000;143(6):755–60.

9. Haciyanli M, Lal G, Morita E, et al. Accuracy of preoperative localization studies and intraoperative parathyroid hormone assay in patients with primary hyperparathyroidism and double adenoma. J Am Coll Surg 2003;197(5):739–46.

10. Sugg SL, Krzywda EA, Demeure MJ, et al. Detection of multiple gland primary hyperparathyroidism in the era of minimally invasive parathyroidectomy. Surgery 2004;136(6):1303–9.

11. Hoang JK, Williams K, Gaillard F, et al. Parathyroid 4D-CT: multi-institutional international survey of use and trends. Otolaryngol Head Neck Surg 2016; 155(6):956–60.

12. Cheung K, Wang TS, Farrokhyar F, et al. A meta-analysis of preoperative localization techniques for patients with primary hyperparathyroidism. Ann Surg Oncol 2012;19(2):577–83.

13. Lubitz CC, Stephen AE, Hodin RA, et al. Preoperative localization strategies for primary hyperparathyroidism: an economic analysis. Ann Surg Oncol 2012;19(13):4202–9.

14. Grimelius L, Bondeson L. Histopathological diagnosis of parathyroid diseases. Pathol Res Pract 1995;191(4):353–65.

15. Akerström G, Malmaeus J, Bergström R. Surgical anatomy of human parathyroid glands. Surgery 1984;95(1):14–21.

16. Mohebati A, AR Shaha. Anatomy of thyroid and parathyroid glands and neurovascular relations. Clinical Anatomy 2011;25(1):19-31.

17. Untch BR, Adam MA, Scheri RP, et al. Surgeon-performed ultrasound is superior to 99Tc-sestamibi scanning to localize parathyroid adenomas in patients with primary hyperparathyroidism: results in 516 patients over 10 years. J Am Coll Surg 2011;212(4):522–9.

18. Lane M, Desser T, Weigel R, et al. Use of color and power Doppler sonography to identify feeding arteries associated with parathyroid adenomas. AJR Am J Roentgenol 1998;171(3):819–23.

19. Reeder SB, Desser TS, Weigel RJ, et al. Sonography in primary hyperparathyroidism: review with emphasis on scanning technique. J Ultrasound Med 2002;21(5): 539–52.

20. Ozturk A, Grajo JR, Dhyani M, et al. Principles of ultrasound elastography. Abdom Radiol (NY) 2018; 43(4):773–85.

21. Batur A, Atmaca M, Yavuz A, et al. Ultrasound elastography for distinction between parathyroid adenomas and thyroid nodules. J Ultrasound Med 2016;35(6):1277–82.

22. Frank SJ, Goldman-Yassen AE, Koenigsberg T, et al. Sensitivity of 3-dimensional sonography in preoperative evaluation of parathyroid glands in patients with primary hyperparathyroidism. J Ultrasound Med 2017;36(9):1897–904.

23. Smith JR, Oates ME. Radionuclide imaging of the parathyroid glands: patterns, pearls, and pitfalls. Radiographics 2004;24(4):1101–15.

24. Zafereo M, Yu J, Angelos P, et al. American Head and Neck Society Endocrine Surgery Section update on parathyroid imaging for surgical candidates with primary hyperparathyroidism. Head Neck 2019; 41(7):2398–409.

25. Biersack H-J, Heiden U. Parathyroid imaging. 99mTc-Sestamibi. Berlin (Germany): Springer; 2012. p. 31–63.

26. Kuzminski SJ, Sosa JA, Hoang JK. Update in parathyroid imaging. Magn Reson Imaging Clin 2018; 26(1):151–66.

27. Rubello D, Massaro A, Cittadin S, et al. Role of 99m Tc-sestamibi SPECT in accurate selection of primary hyperparathyroid patients for minimally invasive radio-guided surgery. Eur J Nucl Med Mol Imaging 2006;33(9):1091–4.

28. Civelek AC, Ozalp E, Donovan P, et al. Prospective evaluation of delayed technetium-99m sestamibi SPECT scintigraphy for preoperative localization of primary hyperparathyroidism. Surgery 2002;131(2): 149–57.

29. Orevi M, Freedman N, Mishani E, et al. Localization of parathyroid adenoma by 11C-choline PET/CT: preliminary results. Clin Nucl Med 2014;39(12): 1033–8.

30. Rep S, Lezaic L, Kocjan T, et al. Optimal scan time for evaluation of parathyroid adenoma with [18F]-fluorocholine PET/CT. Radiol Oncol 2015;49(4): 327–33.

31. Pfob CH, Karimov I, Jesinghaus M, et al. Pitfalls in Ga-68-PSMA-PET/CT: incidental finding of parathyroid adenoma. Eur J Nucl Med Mol Imaging 2019; 46(4):1041.

32. Kelly H, Hamberg L, Hunter G. 4D-CT for preoperative localization of abnormal parathyroid glands in patients with hyperparathyroidism: accuracy and ability to stratify patients by unilateral versus bilateral disease in surgery-naive and re-exploration patients. AJNR Am J Neuroradiol 2014;35(1):176-81.

33. Chazen J, Gupta A, Dunning A, et al. Diagnostic accuracy of 4D-CT for parathyroid adenomas and hyperplasia. AJNR Am J Neuroradiol 2012;33(3): 429–33.

34. Rodgers SE, Hunter GJ, Hamberg LM, et al. Improved preoperative planning for directed parathyroidectomy with 4-dimensional computed tomography. Surgery 2006;140(6):932–41.

35. Harari A, Zarnegar R, Lee J, et al. Computed tomography can guide focused exploration in select patients with primary hyperparathyroidism and negative sestamibi scanning. Surgery 2008;144(6):970–7.

36. Kukar M, Platz TA, Schaffner TJ, et al. The use of modified four-dimensional computed tomography in patients with primary hyperparathyroidism: an argument for the abandonment of routine sestamibi single-positron emission computed tomography (SPECT). Ann Surg Oncol 2015;22(1):139–45.

37. Hinson AM, Lee DR, Hobbs BA, et al. Preoperative 4D CT localization of nonlocalizing parathyroid adenomas by ultrasound and SPECT-CT. Otolaryngol Head Neck Surg 2015;153(5):775–8.

38. Yeh R, Tay Y-KD, Tabacco G, et al. Diagnostic performance of 4D CT and sestamibi SPECT/CT in localizing parathyroid adenomas in primary hyperparathyroidism. Radiology 2019;291(2):469–76.

39. Mortenson MM, Evans DB, Lee JE, et al. Parathyroid exploration in the reoperative neck: improved preoperative localization with 4D-computed tomography. J Am Coll Surg 2008;206(5):888–95.

40. Cham S, Sepahdari AR, Hall KE, et al. Dynamic parathyroid computed tomography (4DCT) facilitates reoperative parathyroidectomy and enables cure of missed hyperplasia. Ann Surg Oncol 2015; 22(11):3537–42.

41. Galvin L, Oldan JD, Bahl M, et al. Parathyroid 4D CT and scintigraphy: what factors contribute to missed parathyroid lesions? Otolaryngol Head Neck Surg 2016;154(5):847–53.

42. Starker LF, Mahajan A, Björklund P, et al. 4D parathyroid CT as the initial localization study for patients with de novo primary hyperparathyroidism. Ann Surg Oncol 2011;18(6):1723–8.

43. Linda DD, Ng B, Rebello R, et al. The utility of multidetector computed tomography for detection of parathyroid disease in the setting of primary hyperparathyroidism. Can Assoc Radiol J 2012;63(2): 100–8.

44. Gafton A, Glastonbury C, Eastwood J, et al. Parathyroid lesions: characterization with dual-phase arterial and venous enhanced CT of the neck. AJNR Am J Neuroradiol 2012;33(5):949–52.

45. Noureldine SI, Aygun N, Walden MJ, et al. Multiphase computed tomography for localization of parathyroid disease in patients with primary hyperparathyroidism: how many phases do we really need? Surgery 2014;156(6):1300–7.

46. Doppman JL, Hammond WG, Melson GL, et al. Staining of parathyroid adenomas by selective arteriography. Radiology 1969;92(3):527–30.

47. Lee EK, Yun TJ, Kim J-h, et al. Effect of tumor volume on the enhancement pattern of parathyroid adenoma on parathyroid four-dimensional CT. Neuroradiology 2016;58(5):495–501.

48. Bahl M, Sepahdari AR, Sosa JA, et al. Parathyroid adenomas and hyperplasia on four-dimensional CT scans: three patterns of enhancement relative to the thyroid gland justify a three-phase protocol. Radiology 2015;277(2):454–62.

49. Kluijfhout WP, Pasternak JD, Beninato T, et al. Diagnostic performance of computed tomography for parathyroid adenoma localization; a systematic review and meta-analysis. Eur J Radiol 2017;88: 117–28.

50. Leiva-Salinas C, Flors L, Durst CR, et al. Detection of parathyroid adenomas using a monophasic dual-energy computed tomography acquisition: diagnostic performance and potential radiation dose reduction. Neuroradiology 2016;58(11):1135–41.

51. Newton T, Eisenberg E. Angiography of parathyroid adenomas. Radiology 1966;86(5):843–50.

52. Bahl M, Muzaffar M, Vij G, et al. Prevalence of the polar vessel sign in parathyroid adenomas on the arterial phase of 4D CT. AJNR Am J Neuroradiol 2014;35(3):578–81.

53. Hoang JK, Sung W-k, Bahl M, et al. How to perform parathyroid 4D CT: tips and traps for technique and interpretation. Radiology 2014;270(1):15–24.

54. Sepahdari A, Bahl M, Harari A, et al. Predictors of multigland disease in primary hyperparathyroidism: a scoring system with 4D-CT imaging and biochemical markers. AJNR Am J Neuroradiol 2015;36(5): 987–92.

55. Sho S, Yilma M, Yeh M, et al. Prospective validation of two 4D-CT–based scoring systems for prediction of multigland disease in primary hyperparathyroidism. AJNR Am J Neuroradiol 2016;37(12):2323–7.

56. Yeh R, Tay Y-K, Dercle L, et al. A simple formula to estimate parathyroid weight on 4D-CT, predict pathologic weight, and diagnose parathyroid adenoma in patients with primary hyperparathyroidism. AJNR Am J Neuroradiol 2020;41(9):1690–7.

57. Mahajan A, Starker LF, Ghita M, et al. Parathyroid four-dimensional computed tomography: evaluation of radiation dose exposure during preoperative localization of parathyroid tumors in primary hyperparathyroidism. World J Surg 2012;36(6):1335–9.

58. Ishibashi M, Nishida H, Hiromatsu Y, et al. Comparison of technetium-99m-MIBI, technetium-99m-tetrofosmin, ultrasound and MRI for localization of abnormal parathyroid glands. J Nucl Med 1998; 39(2):320–4.

59. Lee JC, Kim JS, Lee JH, et al. F-18 FDG-PET as a routine surveillance tool for the detection of recurrent head and neck squamous cell carcinoma. Oral Oncol 2007;43(7):686–92.

60. McDermott V, Fernandez R, Meakem T 3rd, et al. Preoperative MR imaging in hyperparathyroidism: results and factors affecting parathyroid detection. AJR Am J Roentgenol 1996;166(3):705–10.

61. Hänninen EL, Vogl TJ, Steinmüller T, et al. Preoperative contrast-enhanced MRI of the parathyroid glands in hyperparathyroidism. Invest Radiol 2000; 35(7):426–30.

62. Gotway MB, Reddy GP, Webb WR, et al. Comparison between MR imaging and 99mTc MIBI scintigraphy in the evaluation of recurrent or persistent hyperparathyroidism. Radiology 2001;218(3): 783–90.

63. Grayev AM, Gentry LR, Hartman MJ, et al. Presurgical localization of parathyroid adenomas with magnetic resonance imaging at 3.0 T: an adjunct method to supplement traditional imaging. Ann Surg Oncol 2012;19(3):981–9.

64. Kabala J. Computed tomography and magnetic resonance imaging in diseases of the thyroid and parathyroid. Eur J Radiol 2008;66(3):480–92.

65. Sacconi B, Argirò R, Diacinti D, et al. MR appearance of parathyroid adenomas at 3 T in patients with primary hyperparathyroidism: what radiologists

need to know for pre-operative localization. Eur Radiol 2016;26(3):664–73.

66. Argirò R, Diacinti D, Sacconi B, et al. Diagnostic accuracy of 3T magnetic resonance imaging in the preoperative localisation of parathyroid adenomas: comparison with ultrasound and 99mTc-sestamibi scans. Eur Radiol 2018;28(11):4900–8.

67. Merchavy S, Luckman J, Guindy M, et al. 4D MRI for the localization of parathyroid adenoma: a novel method in evolution. Otolaryngol Head Neck Surg 2016;154(3):446–8.

68. Ozturk M, Polat AV, Celenk C, et al. The diagnostic value of 4D MRI at 3T for the localization of parathyroid adenomas. Eur J Radiol 2019;112:207–13.

69. Turski PA, Korosec FR, Carroll TJ, et al. Contrast-enhanced magnetic resonance angiography of the carotid bifurcation using the time-resolved imaging of contrast kinetics (TRICKS) technique. Top Magn Reson Imaging 2001;12(3):175–81.

70. Aschenbach R, Tuda S, Lamster E, et al. Dynamic magnetic resonance angiography for localization of hyperfunctioning parathyroid glands in the reoperative neck. Eur J Radiol 2012;81(11):3371–7.

71. Nael K, Hur J, Bauer A, et al. Dynamic 4D MRI for characterization of parathyroid adenomas: multi-parametric analysis. AJNR Am J Neuroradiol 2015; 36(11):2147–52.

72. Becker J, Patel V, Johnson K, et al. 4D–dynamic contrast-enhanced MRI for preoperative localization in patients with primary hyperparathyroidism. AJNR Am J Neuroradiol 2020;41(3):522–8.

73. Aygün N, Uludağ M. Intraoperative adjunct methods for localization in primary hyperparathyroidism. Sisli Etfal Hastan Tip Bul 2019;53(2):84–95.

Parathyroid Surgery
What Radiologists Need to Know

Aditya S. Shirali, MD, Uriel Clemente-Gutierrez, MD, Nancy D. Perrier, MD*

KEYWORDS

- Hypercalcemia • Hyperparathyroidism • Parathyroidectomy • Localization • Parathyroid carcinoma

KEY POINTS

- Hyperparathyroidism is characterized by hyperfunction of the parathyroid glands resulting in hypercalcemia and a myriad of clinical symptoms.
- Surgical treatment is the only definitive intervention for primary hyperparathyroidism, with surgical options including minimally invasive parathyroidectomy, bilateral cervical exploration, and, in the uncommon event of parathyroid carcinoma, en bloc resection.
- Surgeons use the patient's history and radiographic localization to help determine the operative approach, with a combination of ultrasonography, four-dimensional computed tomography, and Tc99-sestamibi for parathyroid localization.
- An anatomic nomenclature (Perrier parathyroid positions) provides a means to communicate the location of parathyroid glands across multidisciplinary teams to help inform surgical decision making in the initial or reoperative setting.
- Surgical management of hyperparathyroidism is associated with high rates of cure and low rates of persistence or recurrence.

INTRODUCTION

The parathyroid glands play a fundamental role in bone mineral homeostasis. Parathyroid hormone (PTH) regulates serum calcium levels by controlling the rate of bone resorption and the renal tubular handling of calcium and phosphorus. Calcium sensor receptors are expressed in parathyroid and renal tissue. These sensors allow the parathyroid glands to detect the ionized calcium concentration in the extracellular fluid. Normal function of the calcium sensor is critical to calcium reabsorption by the kidney and is also influenced by vitamin D and serum phosphorus levels (Fig. 1).

Hyperparathyroidism (HPT) is an endocrine disease associated with hyperfunction of the parathyroid glands. Multidisciplinary work-up and evaluation is essential in order to offer appropriate treatment of this condition. This multidisciplinary team should include endocrinologists, surgeons, pathologists, and neuroradiologists with special interest in thyroid and parathyroid disorders.

DIAGNOSIS OF HYPERPARATHYROIDISM

HPT is most commonly associated with autonomous hyperfunction of the parathyroid glands, known as primary HPT (PHPT). Prolonged systemic stimulation of the parathyroid glands, as seen in vitamin D deficiency, intestinal malabsorption, or chronic kidney disease, may also lead to parathyroid hyperfunction in a process known as secondary HPT. Tertiary HPT occurs in the setting of renal transplant in patients with prolonged secondary HPT. After receiving a renal allograft, these patients continue to have increased PTH secondary to the long-standing parathyroid stimulation causing autonomous functioning of the parathyroid gland.

PHPT is an endocrine disorder caused by parathyroid adenoma or hyperplastic glands, causing inappropriate increase of serum calcium and PTH levels with systemic manifestations. It is a common endocrine disease and has an estimated prevalence of 0.23% among women and 0.085%

Department of Surgical Oncology, The University of Texas MD Anderson Cancer Center, 1400 Pressler Street, Unit 1484, PO Box 301402, Houston, TX 77030-4009, USA
* Corresponding author.
E-mail address: nperrier@mdanderson.org

Neuroimag Clin N Am 31 (2021) 397–408
https://doi.org/10.1016/j.nic.2021.04.011
1052-5149/21/© 2021 Elsevier Inc. All rights reserved.

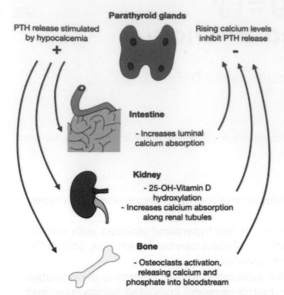

Parathyroid glands

PTH release stimulated by hypocalcemia +

Rising calcium levels inhibit PTH release −

Intestine
- Increases luminal calcium absorption

Kidney
- 25-OH-Vitamin D hydroxylation
- Increases calcium absorption along renal tubules

Bone
- Osteoclasts activation, releasing calcium and phosphate into bloodstream

Fig. 1. The role of parathyroid glands in bone mineral homeostasis.

among men.[1] This endocrine disease can occur as a sporadic entity, accounting for most cases (80%–95%), or associated with different familial disorders (5%–10%) such as multiple endocrine neoplasia (MEN) types 1, 2A, or 4; familial PHPT; and HPT–jaw tumor syndrome.[2] Secondary HPT is common among patients with chronic kidney disease, affecting up to 90% of these patients,[3] whereas tertiary HPT has a reported prevalence of 30% among renal transplant patients.[4]

Clinical Manifestations

Even though classic objective symptoms of PHPT include osteoporosis, nephrolithiasis, gastrointestinal alterations, and pancreatitis, the subjective symptoms are most common and most difficult to quantify. These symptoms include arthralgias, myalgias, and neuropsychiatric symptoms. Because these symptoms cannot be easily measured, the medical misnomer of asymptomatic HPT is sometimes used to describe disease presentation. The diagnosis is usually suspected in the context of the incidental finding of a high normal or increased serum calcium concentration obtained incidentally. Symptoms of profound hypercalcemia, usually more than 14 mg/dL, may include nausea, vomiting, pancreatitis, or coma.[5] Notwithstanding parathyroid carcinoma, this increase occurs slowly over time and is not usually acute.

Unlike PHPT, patients with untreated secondary HPT develop progressive bone disease associated with bone pain, osteitis fibrosa cystica, and soft tissue calcifications. In tertiary HPT, symptoms are similar to patients with severe manifestations of PHPT in addition to the increased risk of worsening renal allograft function.

Biochemical Profile

HPT is a biochemical diagnosis. The initial assessment includes serum calcium level, ionized calcium, phosphorus, creatinine, albumin, PTH, 25-OH vitamin D, bone turnover markers, and 24-hour urinary calcium excretion.

As mentioned previously, in PHPT there is an impaired negative feedback loop between serum calcium and PTH levels. Some variants of PHPT have been described and refer to the group of patients that do not match the classic definition of PHPT. Eucalcemic PHPT is a variant of PHPT usually found in patients who are being evaluated for low bone mineral density, at which time they are found with increased serum PTH level in the absence of hypercalcemia. The diagnosis of this entity should be considered after all causes of secondary HPT have been excluded.[1] Another recognized variant of PHPT is that with normal PTH levels. In this group of patients, increased serum calcium levels are detected, but PTH levels are found within the normal range (ie, an inappropriately normal PTH level).[6]

The biochemical profile of secondary HPT may reveal hypocalcemia or eucalcemia, hyperphosphatemia, extremely increased PTH level, and low vitamin D levels. These findings differ from those seen in tertiary HPT, where serum calcium level is increased accompanied by increased PTH level, hyperphosphatemia, and low vitamin D level (**Table 1**).[7]

Familial Syndromes

Eighty percent of PHPT cases are associated with single parathyroid disease (adenoma). Fifteen percent of PHPT is represented by multigland disease, most commonly seen in familial forms of PHPT. These forms include hereditary diseases such as MEN1, MEN2A, and MEN4, neonatal severe HPT, HPT–jaw tumor syndrome, familial isolated HPT, or autosomal dominant moderate HPT.[8] Familial forms of PHPT must be suspected in patients (1) less than 40 years of age, (2) with other endocrine tumors, and (3) with evidence of multigland disease or parathyroid carcinoma. These patients are referred for genetic counseling.

It is imperative for endocrine surgeons to consider and diagnose familial forms of PHPT, because the work-up and treatment of HPT differ from nonfamilial PHPT, as mentioned later. These patients require specific surveillance for other endocrine tumors and for recurrence of PHPT.

Table 1
Diagnostic test results among different hyperparathyroidism types

Laboratory Test	PHPT	Secondary HPT	Tertiary HPT
Total calcium	↑	↓	↑
Ionized calcium	↑	↓	↑
Phosphorus	↓	↑	↑
Vitamin D	↑	↓	↓
PTH	↑	↑↑	↑↑
Creatinine	N	↑	N

Indications for Operative Management

Surgical treatment is the only definitive intervention for PHPT. Parathyroidectomy is indicated in all symptomatic patients (objective symptoms) with PHPT. For those asymptomatic patients (ie, most patients), surgical treatment is offered according to the Fourth International Workshop Guidelines and American Association of Endocrine Surgeons (AAES) guidelines (**Box 1**).[9,10]

Secondary and tertiary HPT can have benefits from parathyroidectomy as well, although medical treatment should be offered as first line.[11,12] The indications for surgical treatment in these variants of HPT are summarized in **Box 2**.

PREOPERATIVE ASSESSMENT
Clinical History and Examination

Before surgical intervention, the surgeon must obtain a detailed clinical history as outlined later (**Box 3**). Any suggestion of an endocrine syndrome with primary HPT at or before the age of 40 years should prompt genetic counseling and testing.[13] It is crucial that an endocrine surgeon rules out concomitant thyroid disorder preoperatively. Patients found with suspicious thyroid nodules on ultrasonography (US) should prompt fine-needle aspiration (FNA) for cytologic assessment and, if deemed necessary, undergo concomitant thyroid resection to prevent reoperative neck surgery.

Detailed surgical and oncologic histories focusing on prior malignancies and neck or chest operations should be reviewed. If present, all information regarding interventions should be sought. Routine preoperative laryngoscopy in asymptomatic patients adds to overall health care expenses without significant benefit.[14] It is our practice that patients with previous thyroid or parathyroid surgery or voice changes receive preoperative videostroboscopy.[10] A study using the Collaborative Endocrine Surgery Quality Improvement Program found that less than 50% of surgeons used preoperative laryngoscopy in reoperative parathyroidectomy with less than

1% risk of recurrent laryngeal nerve injury,[15] which highlights the importance of preoperative patient screening.

Parathyroid carcinoma should be suspected in the setting of marked hypercalcemia (≥14 mg/dL), PTH 3 to 4 times greater than normal levels or in the presence of a palpable, firm, or fixed cervical mass.[13] These patients require en bloc resection of the involved parathyroid gland, ipsilateral thyroid lobectomy, and surrounding lymphatic tissue.

Preoperative Noninvasive and Invasive Radiography

Preoperative localization of abnormal parathyroid glands is essential for minimally invasive parathyroidectomy (MIP). Technitium-99m sestamibi and parathyroid US are the most commonly used localization studies.[16] The primary techniques for preoperative localization at our institution include some combination of US, sestamibi, and/or four-dimensional (4D) computed tomography (CT).[17] These are discussed in a previous article in this issue.

Ultrasonography plays a key role because of its cost-effectiveness and added benefit of

---

Box 1
Indications for surgical treatment of asymptomatic patients

- Serum calcium level more than 1 mg/dL greater than the upper limit of normal
- Osteoporosis
- Vertebral fracture documented by imaging studies
- Creatinine clearance less than 60 mL/min
- Twenty-four-hour urine calcium level greater than 400 mg/dL (>10 mmol/dL)
- Nephrolithiasis or nephrocalcinosis
- Age less than 50 years

Box 2
Indications for parathyroidectomy in secondary and tertiary hyperparathyroidism

Secondary HPT	Tertiary HPT
• Calciphylaxis	• Severe hypercalcemia (serum calcium >11.5 mg/dL)
• Patient preference	
• Medical observation not possible	• Persistent hypercalcemia >3 mo to 1 y after transplant
• Failure of maximal medical management associated with:	• Severe osteopenia
	• Symptomatic HPT:
○ Hypercalcemia	○ Fatigue
○ Hypercalciuria	○ Pruritus
○ PTH>800 pg/mL	○ Bone pain or pathologic bone fracture
○ Hyperphosphatemia	
○ Osteoporosis	○ Peptic ulcer disease
○ Untreatable symptoms: pruritus, pathologic bone fracture, ectopic soft tissue calcifications, severe vascular calcifications, bone pain	○ Mental status changes
	○ History of renal calculi

Modified from Pitt SC, Sippel RS, Chen H. Secondary and tertiary hyperparathyroidism, state of the art surgical management. *Surg Clin North Am.* 2009;89(5):1227-1239.

---

identifying any concomitant thyroid disorder. The authors routinely perform US from the submandibular region cephalad to the clavicles caudally with the addition of Doppler imaging to assess the vascularity of any suspicious lesions and inform the surgeon of the vascular pedicle, which may be important with regard to decision making for operative approach and angles of dissection for limited manipulation of surrounding tissue. Given the occasional failure of ultrasonographic identification of parathyroid adenomas, the authors recommend the use of planar sestamibi imaging and 4D-CT because it offers the highest sensitivity for localization of hyperfunctioning parathyroid glands.[17]

Radiographic identification of pathologic parathyroid glands in candidates for parathyroid reoperation is key to surgical success. Sometimes noninvasive studies do not clearly identify an adenoma. Before considering invasive testing such as arterial or venous sampling, US-guided parathyroid FNA with PTH washout may be considered. In a study performed at the Mayo Clinic, Bancos and colleagues[18] found that parathyroid FNA with PTH washout had a sensitivity of 84%, specificity of 100%, and accuracy of 84% with 6.7% of patients who eventually went on to a focus

parathyroidectomy requiring conversion to bilateral cervical exploration because of complications from aspirate. When parathyroid carcinoma is considered, FNA or core biopsy should be avoided because of possible needle tracking of tumor.[19,20] En bloc resection offers the best chance of cure, and tumor seeding and local recurrence can be biochemically fatal because the patient demise is from malignant hypercalcemia.

Box 3
Clinical history

- History of pituitary adenomas or duodeno-pancreatic neuroendocrine tumors (MEN1), medullary thyroid cancer or pheochromocytoma (MEN2A), or mandibular tumors (HPT–jaw tumor syndrome)
- Family history of HPT and other endocrinopathies
- Concomitant thyroid disorder
- History of neck radiation
- Detailed surgical and oncologic history (previous thyroid, parathyroid, or other neck operations)

Parathyroid Nomenclature System

The authors have developed a nomenclature system based on the most frequently encountered positions of enlarged parathyroid glands and use this to communicate the location of the suspected abnormal gland between our surgeons and radiologists, anesthesiologists, pathologists, and endocrinologists (Fig. 2).[21] Superior and inferior glands are defined by the location of the gland's pedicle and its relationship to the recurrent laryngeal nerve. Superior glands anatomically have a vascular pedicle superior and lateral to the recurrent laryngeal nerve (type A through D glands). Inferior glands have a vascular pedicle inferior and medial to the recurrent laryngeal nerve (type D through F glands). Type G glands represent intrathyroidal parathyroid lesions and type H glands are rare and halfway between left and right, residing in the posterior esophageal midline.[22] This information helps surgeons to know how to proceed with dissection near the nerve, especially when a limited approach may not allow early identification of the nerve in the tracheoesophageal groove.

Approach to Operative Selection

As outlined earlier, patients who are diagnosed with biochemical HPT require an extensive discussion regarding their prior familial and surgical histories in addition to preoperative physical examination and laboratory assessment to help determine operative approach. Fig. 3 outlines our algorithm for selecting patients for MIP, bilateral cervical exploration, or discussion of en bloc resection because of concern for parathyroid carcinoma. In the reoperative parathyroidectomy, review of prior operative and pathology reports in addition to concomitant concordant imaging or preoperative confirmative PTH FNA is necessary.

SURGICAL MANAGEMENT OF HYPERPARATHYROIDISM

The success rate of operative treatment of PHPT is higher than 95%, and morbidity is seen in less than

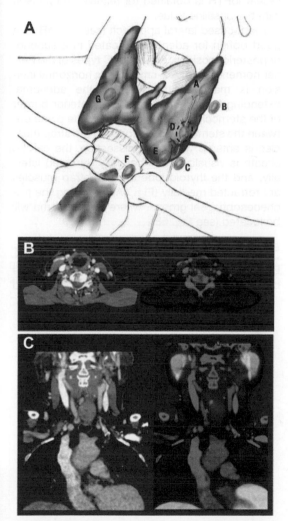

Fig. 2. (A) Perrier nomenclature for adenomatous parathyroid glands A to G. (B and C) Type H glands denoted by blue arrows identified in the midline posterior to the esophagus on sestamibi single-photon emission CT/CT imaging in (B) axial and (C) coronal imaging planes. (From Gallagher JW, Kelley ML, Yip L, Carty SE, McCoy KL. Retropharyngeal Parathyroid Glands: Important Differences. *World J Surg.* 2018;42(2):437-443.)

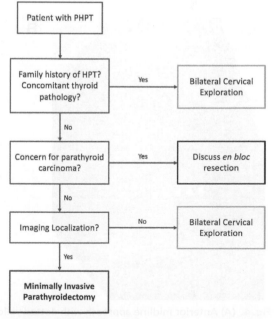

Fig. 3. Algorithm for surgical intervention selection.

1% of patients.[23,24] The options of surgical treatment of HPT depend on the nature of the disease. In patients with PHPT, where the most common cause is a single adenoma in 80% to 85%, a MIP may be an adequate option with appropriate preoperative assessment and localization studies. In contrast, patients with multigland disease (either sporadic or associated with familial PHPT), secondary or tertiary HPT require bilateral cervical exploration for durable cure.

Minimally Invasive Parathyroidectomy

MIP is an excellent option for the treatment of PHPT. The advantages of MIP include smaller incision, lower complication rate, shorter operative time, lower cost, less postoperative pain, the possibility of same-day discharge, and (most importantly) a cure rate that is comparable with bilateral cervical exploration.[24]

It must be emphasized that MIP currently requires preoperative radiographic localization to suggest where to start and intraoperative PTH monitoring (ioPTH) to facilitate decision making, when necessary, of when to stop. Multiple criteria have been described to determine the success of the operation. The most commonly used protocol is a greater than 50% decrease from the highest preincision ioPTH level relative to a 5-minute or 10-minute postexcision ioPTH level after excision of hyperfunctioning parathyroid tissue.[25] Different surgical approaches based on enlarged gland location include the anterior midline and focused lateral approaches. Both techniques are performed with the patient placed in semi-Fowler position with delicate neck extension.

On the anterior midline approach (**Fig. 4**A), a 2-cm to 3-cm horizontal incision is made 1 cm below the cricoid cartilage. The strap muscles are separated in the midline and with blunt dissection the thyroid is separated from the overlying muscles. Medial retraction of the thyroid lobe simplifies exposure of the enlarged gland. Once the enlarged gland is localized, it has to be dissected from the surrounding tissue, the vascular pedicle is ligated, and the gland excised. After a 5-minute to 10-minute waiting period to allow a decline in PTH levels, repeat ioPTH is obtained for relative comparison with the baseline value.

The focused lateral approach (see **Fig. 4**B) is a good option for adenomas located in a superior or posterior position, or A, B, or C types of the Perrier nomenclature. A 2-cm to 3-cm horizontal incision is made at the level of the adenoma, extending from the midline to the anterior border of the sternocleidomastoid muscle. The plane between the sternocleidomastoid and the strap muscles is entered with blunt dissection, the carotid sheath is visualized and carefully retracted laterally, and the thyroid lobe and the strap muscles are retracted medially (**Fig. 5**A), exposing the tracheoesophageal groove, where the adenoma will be located (see **Fig. 5**B).

Bilateral Cervical Exploration

Bilateral cervical exploration is intended to explore both sides of the neck and identify the 4 parathyroid

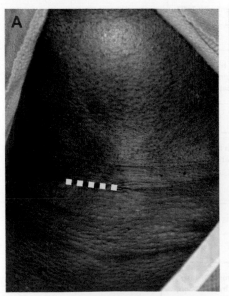 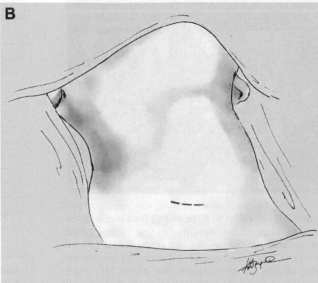

Fig. 4. (*A*) Anterior midline approach with dotted yellow line representing incision. (*B*) Focused lateral approach with dotted black line representing incision.

glands. This approach is recommended for patients with negative or discordant preoperative imaging for which the chance of single-gland disease is lower than 85% (familial PHPT, secondary and tertiary HPT).

The procedure is performed under general anesthesia, with the patient in semi-Fowler position, and with gentle neck extension. A 2-cm to 3-cm horizontal incision is made 1 cm below the cricoid cartilage between both anterior borders of sternocleidomastoid muscles. The strap muscles are separated in the midline and blunt dissection is performed between the thyroid and the strap muscles laterally. The thyroid lobe is medialized and both superior and inferior parathyroid glands are inspected. If an obvious enlarged adenoma is identified, it is excised. If not, all 4 glands are inspected and the largest removed. In patients with sporadic hyperplasia, subtotal resection of the most normal-appearing hyperplastic glands is performed. The parathyroid tissue remnant should be the size of a normal parathyroid gland, approximately 40 to 60 mg. Histology is used to confirm that the tissue is of parathyroid origin.

On confirmation that the remnant is viable, the other abnormal parathyroid glands are resected.

Patients with familial HPT require more nuanced surgical decision making. In contrast with patients with sporadic disease, where solitary adenomas occur in about 80% of cases, more than 80% of patients with familial disease have multiple abnormal glands. Supernumerary glands are also more common. If inadequate removal of hyperfunctioning is performed, recurrence is likely. Subtotal (3.5-gland) parathyroidectomy is the procedure of choice. In light of the advantages of the subtotal parathyroidectomy procedure, the recommendations of tertiary care centers and experts have favored subtotal parathyroidectomy when treating PHPT in patients with MEN1. The goal of this approach is leaving a remnant 1.5 to 2 times the size of a normal gland (40–60 mg). Bilateral cervical thymectomy is also performed in order to identify supernumerary glands and, in men, decrease the risk of thymic carcinoid tumors.[26]

The optimal surgical intervention must balance the risk of recurrent hypercalcemia with the morbidity of permanent hypoparathyroidism. The authors favor subtotal parathyroidectomy over total parathyroidectomy with autotransplant given

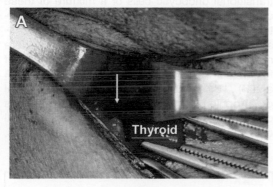

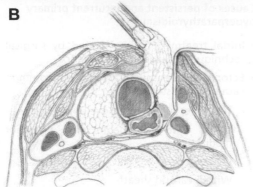

Fig. 5. (A) Retraction of the thyroid lobe medially to expose tracheoesophageal groove. Yellow arrow identifies tracheoesophageal groove. Blue arrow identifies direction of medial retraction. (B) Exposing tracheoesophageal groove to identify types B and C parathyroid adenomas.

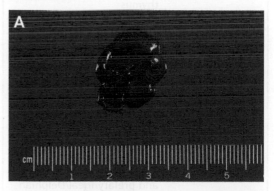

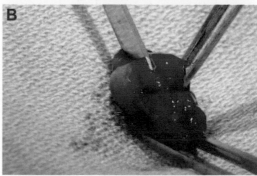

Fig. 6. (A) Parathyroid adenoma before histologic evaluation. (B) Parathyroid adenoma being bivalved immediately after resection.

the significant morbidity associated with permanent hypoparathyroidism.

En Bloc Resection for Parathyroid Carcinoma

Parathyroid carcinoma (PC) is a rare entity, presenting in less than 1% of patients with PHPT.

Table 2 American Joint Committee on Cancer Eighth Edition Staging of Parathyroid Carcinoma	
Primary Tumor (T)	
Tx	Primary tumor cannot be assessed
T0	No evidence of primary tumor
Tis	Atypical parathyroid neoplasm (neoplasm of uncertain malignant potential)[a]
T1	Localized to the parathyroid gland with extension limited to soft tissue
T2	Direct invasion into the thyroid gland
T3	Direct invasion into recurrent laryngeal nerve, esophagus, trachea, skeletal muscle, adjacent lymph nodes, or thymus
T4	Direct invasion into major blood vessel or spine
Regional Lymph Nodes (N)	
NX	Regional nodes cannot be assessed
N0	No regional lymph node metastasis
N1	Regional lymph node metastasis
N1a	Metastasis to level VI (pretracheal, paratracheal, and prelaryngeal/Delphian lymph nodes) or superior mediastinal lymph nodes (level VII)
N1b	Metastasis to unilateral, bilateral, or contralateral cervical (level I, II, III, IV, or V) or retropharyngeal nodes
Distant Metastasis (M)	
cM0	No distant metastasis
cM1	Distant metastasis
pM1	Distant metastasis, microscopically confirmed

[a] Defined as tumors that are histologically or clinically worrisome but do not fulfill the more robust criteria (ie, invasion, metastasis) for carcinoma.

Historically, the clinical presentation has been related to profound hypercalcemia, which may manifest as bone disease, renal disease, or pancreatitis. A painless, subtle neck mass can be palpable at physical examination. Biochemical work-up reveals markedly increased serum calcium and PTH levels. The diagnosis is usually initiated on clinical suspicion and the most common intraoperative findings are local invasion of contiguous structures.[27]

Surgery is the cornerstone in the treatment of PC. En bloc resection has been established as the standard of treatment and it includes performing a parathyroidectomy, ipsilateral thyroid lobectomy, central neck dissection, and, if necessary, resection of the thymus. Factors independently associated with survival were age (hazard ratio [HR], 1.05) and distant metastases (HR, 4.73).[28]

PATHOLOGY

PHPT can be caused by 4 different pathologic lesions: adenoma, hyperplasia, atypical neoplasm, and carcinoma. An adenoma is a benign neoplasm composed primarily of chief cells with occasional transitional oncocytic cells or a mixture of these cell types.[29] Adenomas are macroscopically identified as well-circumscribed, smooth, and occasionally encapsulated lesions and are responsible for approximately 80% of cases of PHPT and usually affect a single gland (**Figs. 6**A and B).[30] By definition, the other glands are normal or atrophic. Primary parathyroid hyperplasia is defined as an absolute increase in parenchymal cell mass, resulting from an increase in chief cells,

---

Box 4
Causes of persistent and recurrent primary hyperparathyroidism

- Initial treatment failure caused by surgical technique or surgeon inexperience
- Ectopic or supernumerary glands (common cause of persistent HPT)
  - Tracheoesophageal groove posteriorly
  - Along the esophagus in posterior mediastinum
  - Intrathyroidal
  - Within carotid sheath
- Biology of disease
  - Sporadic or familial multigland disease
  - Parathyromatosis
  - PC

oncocytic cells, transitional oncocytic cell mixtures, and stromal elements in the absence of a known stimulus, and accounts for approximately 15% of PHPT.[29]

It is possible to determine whether a parathyroid gland is normal or hyperplastic intraoperatively. Hyperplastic or adenomatous glands are darker, firmer, and larger. Most adenomas involve a single gland, whereas 3% to 12% of PHPT has double adenomas and should be considered the exception rather than the rule.[31]

Parathyroid carcinoma and atypical adenomas are responsible for less than 5% of PHPT, with PC being responsible for less than 1% of

PHPT.[32] On histology, both may show fibrosis, nuclear atypia, necrosis, and conspicuous mitotic figures. However, per World Health Organization criteria, PC requires lymphovascular invasion, invasion into adjacent structures, or metastatic disease.[29] The differentiation between the two has been made easier by the use of a diagnostic nomogram using a combination of immunohistochemical biomarkers, which highlights that they represent distinct clinical entities.[33,34] The development of PC is usually sporadic and affects 1 gland; however, certain familial endocrine disorders, such as HPT–jaw tumor syndrome (CDC73 mutation) might be associated with PC.[35]

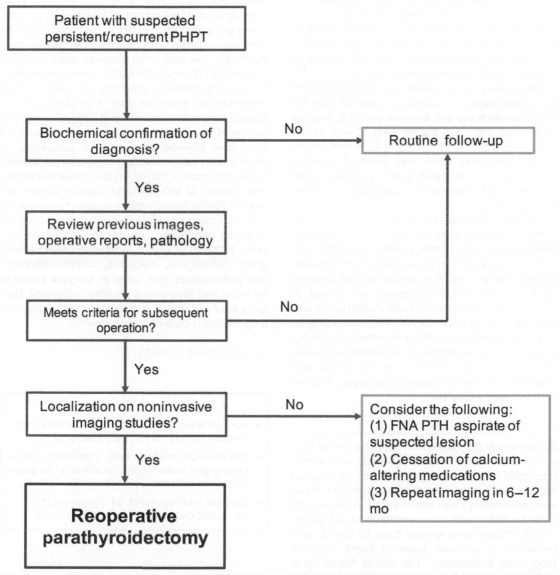

Fig. 7. Algorithm for work-up and management of patients with persistent or recurrent PHPT. (Adapted from Wilhelm SM, Wang TS, Ruan DT, et al. The American Association of Endocrine Surgeons Guidelines for Definitive Management of Primary Hyperparathyroidism. *JAMA Surg.* 2016;151(10):959-968.)

Recently, the American Joint Committee on Cancer (AJCC) Eighth Edition proposed tumor-node-metastasis (TNM) categories for PC (**Table 2**) with distant metastasis as the major predictor of overall survival.[36]

OUTCOMES
Persistent and Recurrent Hyperparathyroidism

Cure rates for sporadic PHPT approach 90% to 95%. A successful parathyroidectomy is defined by normalization of calcium level (and PTH in the event of eucalcemic HPT) at 6 months. Persistent HPT, defined as failure to achieve normocalcemia within 6 months of parathyroidectomy, and recurrent HPT, defined as hypercalcemia after a normocalcemic interval at more than 6 months postoperatively, are rare events in the hands of experienced endocrine surgeons.[15] Our practice is to obtain repeat calcium and PTH levels at 2 weeks and 6 months postoperatively.

The causes of persistent and recurrent PHPT are shown in **Box 4**. Although rates of cure for parathyroidectomy are exceedingly high, studies with longer follow-up are showing 10-year recurrence rates ranging from 10% to 15% with no difference between MIP and bilateral cervical exploration,[37–39] suggesting that patients would benefit from long-term follow-up of their hypercalcemia.

The safest treatment of persistent and recurrent PHPT is avoidance by successful first operation. When approaching management of a patient suspected of persistent and recurrent PHPT, the authors follow an algorithm similar to that outlined by the 2016 AAES guidelines, as shown in **Fig. 7**.[10] After biochemical confirmation of the disease, we review previous records, including prior imaging, operative reports, and pathologic testing. If the patient is considered an operative candidate, we obtain noninvasive imaging with 4D-CT and sestamibi with the intention of identifying a target for a focused exploration.

Parathyroid Carcinoma

As previously discussed, the best chance for cure of PC is complete surgical resection with microscopically negative margins that can be reached with en bloc resection at the first operation. However, recurrence rates are reported to range from 33% to 78%, with age greater than 65 years, serum calcium level greater than 15 mg/dL, and presence of vascular invasion being negative prognostic indicators.[40] The aim of follow-up is early detection of locoregional recurrence and/or metastases. These patients are followed for their lifetimes with biannual serum calcium and PTH levels for the first 5 years, then annually, with annual neck US and/or CT neck. The management of recurrent disease is mainly surgical, and often multiple surgical interventions are performed over time, with the aim being controlling metabolic derangements associated with morbidity rather than complete tumor debulking. Nevertheless, these patients have 5-year and 10-year survival rates of 72% to 85% and 49.1% to 88%, respectively.[41,42] Beyond surgical intervention, few systemic therapies exist to curtail the disease burden.

SUMMARY

HPT is an endocrine disorder associated with hyperfunctioning parathyroid glands with a myriad of symptoms. Most commonly caused by an adenoma or hyperplasia, PHPT is the most common form encountered by clinicians. After biochemical diagnosis, the endocrine surgeon must combine a thorough history with radiographic localization to suggest where to start the operation and to determine an operative plan. If single-gland disease is suspected and imaging suggests concentration of uptake, a MIP is an ideal approach. If multigland disease is present or suspected, a bilateral cervical exploration should be performed. In the rare case of PC, an en bloc resection is recommended. At MD Anderson Cancer Center, we use the Perrier nomenclature system to cohesively communicate to multiple disciplines the location of enlarged parathyroid glands. This approach provides a common language between endocrinologists, radiologists, surgeons, anesthesiologists, and pathologists that helps in surgical planning for initial and reoperative parathyroidectomy. Surgical intervention for parathyroidectomy provides long-standing cure of hypercalcemia.

CLINICS CARE POINTS

- Surgical treatment is the only definitive intervention for primary hyperparathyroidism.
- The surgeon must use both a patient's clinical history and radiographic localization to guide operative approach.
- Surgical management of hyperparathyroidism is associated with high rates of cure.

DISCLOSURES

None.

REFERENCES

1. Dawood NB, Yan KL, Shieh A, et al. Normocalcaemic primary hyperparathyroidism: an update on diagnostic and management challenges. Clin Endocrinol 2020;93(5):519–27.

2. Pepe J, Cipriani C, Pilotto R, et al. Sporadic and hereditary primary hyperparathyroidism. J Endocrinol Invest 2011;34(7 Suppl):40–4.

3. Memmos DE, Williams GB, Eastwood JB, et al. The role of parathyroidectomy in the management of hyperparathyroidism in patients on maintenance haemodialysis and after renal transplantation. Nephron 1982;30(2):143–8.

4. Rivelli GG, Lima MLd, Mazzali M. Therapy for persistent hypercalcemic hyperparathyroidism post-renal transplant: cinacalcet versus parathyroidectomy. J Bras Nefrol 2020;42(3):315–22.

5. Kearns AE, Thompson GB. Medical and surgical management of hyperparathyroidism. Mayo Clin Proc 2002;77(1):87–91.

6. Applewhite MK, Schneider DF. Mild primary hyperparathyroidism: a literature review. Oncologist 2014;19(9):919–29.

7. Pitt SC, Sippel RS, Chen H. Secondary and tertiary hyperparathyroidism, state of the art surgical management. Surg Clin North Am 2009;89(5):1227–39.

8. Brandi ML, Tonelli F. Genetic Syndromes Associated with Primary Hyperparathyroidism. In: Gasparri G, Palestini N, Camandona M, editors. Primary, secondary and tertiary hyperparathyroidism: diagnostic and therapeutic updates. Milano: Springer Milan; 2016. p. 153–81.

9. Bilezikian JP, Brandi ML, Eastell R, et al. Guidelines for the management of asymptomatic primary hyperparathyroidism: summary statement from the fourth international workshop. J Clin Endocrinol Metab 2014;99(10):3561–9.

10. Wilhelm SM, Wang TS, Ruan DT, et al. The American Association of endocrine surgeons guidelines for definitive management of primary hyperparathyroidism. JAMA Surg 2016;151(10):959–68.

11. Yajima A, Ogawa Y, Takahashi HE, et al. Changes of bone remodeling immediately after parathyroidectomy for secondary hyperparathyroidism. Am J Kidney Dis 2003;42(4):729–38.

12. Sharma J, Raggi P, Kutner N, et al. Improved long-term survival of dialysis patients after near-total parathyroidectomy. J Am Coll Surg 2012;214(4):400–7 [discussion 407-8].

13. Zagzag J, Hu MI, Fisher SB, et al. Hypercalcemia and cancer: Differential diagnosis and treatment. CA Cancer J Clin 2018;68(5):377–86.

14. Fowler GE, Chew PR, Lim CBB, et al. Is there a role for routine laryngoscopy before and after parathyroid surgery? Surgeon 2019;17(2):102–6.

15. Kazaure HS, Thomas S, Scheri RP, et al. The devil is in the details: assessing treatment and outcomes of 6,795 patients undergoing remedial parathyroidectomy in the Collaborative Endocrine Surgery Quality Improvement Program. Surgery 2019;165(1):242–9.

16. Siperstein A, Berber E, Mackey R, et al. Prospective evaluation of sestamibi scan, ultrasonography, and rapid PTH to predict the success of limited exploration for sporadic primary hyperparathyroidism. Surgery 2004;136(4):872–80.

17. Rodgers SE, Hunter GJ, Hamberg LM, et al. Improved preoperative planning for directed parathyroidectomy with 4-dimensional computed tomography. Surgery 2006;140(6):932–40 [discussion 940-1].

18. Bancos I, Grant CS, Nadeem S, et al. Risks and benefits of parathyroid fine-needle aspiration with parathyroid hormone washout. Endocr Pract 2012;18(4):441–9.

19. Kim J, Horowitz G, Hong M, et al. The dangers of parathyroid biopsy. J Otolaryngol Head Neck Surg 2017;46(1):4.

20. Spinelli C, Bonadio AG, Berti P, et al. Cutaneous spreading of parathyroid carcinoma after fine needle aspiration cytology. J Endocrinol Invest 2000;23(4):255–7.

21. Perrier ND, Edeiken B, Nunez R, et al. A novel nomenclature to classify parathyroid adenomas. World J Surg 2009;33(3):412–6.

22. Gallagher JW, Kelley ML, Yip L, et al. Retropharyngeal parathyroid glands: important differences. World J Surg 2018;42(2):437–43.

23. Yen TW, Wilson SD, Krzywda EA, et al. The role of parathyroid hormone measurements after surgery for primary hyperparathyroidism. Surgery 2006;140(4):665–72 [discussion 672-664].

24. Udelsman R. Six hundred fifty-six consecutive explorations for primary hyperparathyroidism. Ann Surg 2002;235(5):665–72.

25. Khan ZF, Lew JI. Intraoperative parathyroid hormone monitoring in the surgical management of sporadic primary hyperparathyroidism. Endocrinol Metab (Seoul) 2019;34(4):327–39.

26. Nobecourt PF, Zagzag J, Asare EA, et al. Intraoperative decision-making and technical aspects of parathyroidectomy in young patients with MEN1 related hyperparathyroidism. Front Endocrinol 2018;9:618.

27. Quaglino F, Manfrino L, Cestino L, et al. Parathyroid carcinoma: an up-to-date retrospective multicentric analysis. Int J Endocrinol 2020;2020:7048185.

28. Young S, Wu JX, Li N, et al. More extensive surgery may not improve survival over parathyroidectomy alone in parathyroid carcinoma. Ann Surg Oncol 2016;23(9):2898–904.

29. Guilmette J, Sadow PM. Parathyroid pathology. Surg Pathol Clin 2019;12(4):1007–19.

30. Marcocci C, Cetani F. Clinical practice. Primary hyperparathyroidism. N Engl J Med 2011;365(25):2389–97.

31. Bergson EJ, Heller KS. The clinical significance and anatomic distribution of parathyroid double adenomas. J Am Coll Surg 2004;198(2):185–9.

32. Rodgers SE, Perrier ND. Parathyroid carcinoma. Curr Opin Oncol 2006;18(1):16–22.

33. Christakis I, Bussaidy N, Clarke C, et al. Differentiating atypical parathyroid neoplasm from parathyroid cancer. Ann Surg Oncol 2016;23(9):2889–97.

34. Silva-Figueroa AM, Bassett R Jr, Christakis I, et al. Using a novel diagnostic nomogram to differentiate malignant from benign parathyroid neoplasms. Endocr Pathol 2019;30(4):285–96.

35. Cetani F, Pardi E, Marcocci C. Parathyroid carcinoma. Front Horm Res 2019;51:63–76.

36. Landry CD, Wang TS, Asare EA, et al. Parathyroid. In: Amin MB, editor. AJCC cancer staging manual Eighth edition. New York, NY: Springer International Publishing; 2017. p. 903.

37. Lou I, Balentine C, Clarkson S, et al. How long should we follow patients after apparently curative parathyroidectomy? Surgery 2017;161(1):54–61.

38. Mallick R, Nicholson KJ, Yip L, et al. Factors associated with late recurrence after parathyroidectomy for primary hyperparathyroidism. Surgery 2020;167(1):160–5.

39. Schneider DF, Mazeh H, Chen H, et al. Predictors of recurrence in primary hyperparathyroidism: an analysis of 1386 cases. Ann Surg 2014;259(3):563–8.

40. Silva-Figueroa AM, Hess KR, Williams MD, et al. Prognostic scoring system to risk stratify parathyroid carcinoma. J Am Coll Surg 2017;S1072-7515(17)30179–5.

41. Christakis I, Silva AM, Kwatampora LJ, et al. Oncologic progress for the treatment of parathyroid carcinoma is needed. J Surg Oncol 2016;114(6):708–13.

42. Salcuni AS, Cetani F, Guarnieri V, et al. Parathyroid carcinoma. Best Pract Res Clin Endocrinol Metab 2018;32(6):877–89.

Moving?

Make sure your subscription moves with you!

To notify us of your new address, find your **Clinics Account Number** (located on your mailing label above your name), and contact customer service at:

Email: journalscustomerservice-usa@elsevier.com

800-654-2452 (subscribers in the U.S. & Canada)
314-447-8871 (subscribers outside of the U.S. & Canada)

Fax number: 314-447-8029

Elsevier Health Sciences Division
Subscription Customer Service
3251 Riverport Lane
Maryland Heights, MO 63043

*To ensure uninterrupted delivery of your subscription, please notify us at least 4 weeks in advance of move.

Printed and bound by CPI Group (UK) Ltd, Croydon, CR0 4YY

03/10/2024

01040307-0016